FREEDOM FROM ARTHRITIS

THROUGH

NUTRITION

A Guidebook for Pain-Free Living
With Original Recipes
Expanded, Sixth Edition

PHILIP J. WELSH, D.D.S., N. D.
and
BIANCA LEONARDO, N. D.

Foreword by Robert S. Mendelsohn, M.D.

Tree of Life Publications

Freedom from Arthritis through Nutrition
© Copyright, 1992, Tree of Life Publications

Tree of Life Publications
P. O. Box 126
Joshua Tree, CA 92252

Sixth Edition, updated, 1992
10 9 8 7 6
ISBN: 0-930852-15-X

Library of Congress Cataloging-in-Publication Data

Welsh, Philip.
    Freedom from arthritis through nutrition: a guidebook for pain-free living with original recipes / Philip J. Welsh and Bianca Leonardo. Foreword by Robert S. Mendelsohn. -- 6th ed., updated.
            p.   cm.
    Includes references and index.
    ISBN 0-930852-15-X
    1. Arthritis--Diet therapy. 2. Arthritis--Nutritional aspects.
3. Naturopathy.   I. Leonardo, Bianca II. Title.
RC933.W44   1992
616.7'220654--dc20
                                                          92-9274
                                                          CIP

DEDICATION

This manual is dedicated with compassion to the *millions* of persons who are suffering *needlessly* from arthritis and other diseases, who have lost their way from the path of natural living.

It is also dedicated to the *thousands* of persons who have already found their way back through this revolutionary plan using natural methods, and found freedom from pain and renewed health and life.

P.J.W. and B.A.L.

ACKNOWLEDGEMENT

By the time the first three editions of our book, *How to Be Free From Arthritis Pain* were sold out, we were deeply impressed with and saddened by the amount and severity of suffering that arthritis is causing. We have letters from persons all over the nation telling us of their severe suffering.

Many of these sufferers who have tried to get relief from drugs but failed are very glad to learn of a *harmless, more natural, nutritional* method of helping to combat arthritis. The many grateful letters we have received from readers of our book indicate that the information we are broadcasting is of real help. We wish to thank these readers for taking the time to send us their many grateful letters. A few are included in this book.

DISCLAIMER

The information in this book is intended to describe a particular plan that some arthritis sufferers have adopted, with good results. It is not intended to replace the services of a competent health practitioner.

Neither the authors nor the publisher claim that this book and the plan contained therein, is a remedy for any condition, disease or malfunction of the human body, including arthritis, nor do they promise that users of this method will receive any benefit from following it.

However, the authors and publisher have received letters from people who have purchased this book, tried the plan and received help in the relief of arthritis miseries. In some cases, persons claim extraordinary results.

Experience has taught us that it is more prudent to make lesser claims and deliver better results than to make greater claims and deliver less satisfactory results.

Real joy does not come from ease or riches, but from doing something worthwhile for others on this same earth trip we all are on. There is nothing more worthwhile than helping sick people regain their health, for it is truly said, "Health is Wealth."

A PERSONAL MESSAGE FROM DR. WELSH TO YOU

Dear Friend:

Before you go any further in reading this book, I would like to give you this message:

You should not look upon this manual as just another ordinary book on arthritis. Here is an entirely new approach to the serious problem of arthritis. It is the culmination of over 50 years of intensive study and much experience, and brings you a simple, natural plan, more in harmony with the workings of the body. Readers of several previous editions of this same book have written telling us of the good results they have obtained.

As you read through the pages, you will realize that every recommendation we make has been thoroughly tested, re-tested, and finally adopted after it proved good and sound. These tests were made not only on many arthritis sufferers but also on my own body.

In 1923, my wife Grace was stricken with a severe case of rheumatoid arthritis. After the treatments of the medical doctors failed to give her any relief, I decided to try *Nutritional Therapy;* I had been specializing in nutrition.

To make a long story short (details follow in the book), *my wife was completely rid of her arthritis pain!*

This made a very deep impression upon me, and I decided to concentrate on the treatment of arthritis with *Nutritional Therapy.* This did not involve the use of any drugs, salves, or gadgets of any kind. It was and is a purely natural approach which is safe, simple, and inexpensive. In fact, users of my plan of nutrition *save money* on grocery bills.

v

An ideal opportunity for me to learn about arthritis presented itself when, many years ago, the medical profession — not knowing the cause of arthritis — blamed it on bad teeth. This caused many patients to be sent to their dentists to have their teeth extracted, with the (vain) hope that this would rid them of the arthritis.

I saw that usually the teeth were in good condition. So, instead of extracting the teeth, I would put the patient on a special diet, and in that way helped many arthritis sufferers get well without losing their teeth unnecessarily.

This manual contains a wealth of practical information that is priceless. *In order to get the most benefit, you should read it several times.*

Now, I realize that some of our readers will find it difficult to carry out the plan in its entirety. If such is the case with you, *do not become discouraged.*

From experience, we have found that even if one only partially works this plan, the results will be very rewarding.

If you will read some of the many reports we have received from readers of this manual, you will note that those who adopted the suggestions therein, not only were helped to overcome arthritis, but were also rewarded with better health in general. Some also lost excess weight.

If you give Nature half a chance it will bless you in many ways. So, just do the best you can under your circumstances, and we can assure you — you will be well pleased with the results.

"More than 37 million Americans suffer from some form of arthritis. There are a hundred-odd forms of the disease, from 'bowler's thumb' and 'tennis elbow' to gout and the great crippler, rheumatoid arthritis. More than 97 percent of individuals past sixty have sufficient arthritis that it can be seen on X-ray studies." (Lawrence E. Lamb, M.D.)

The U.S. News and World Report has called arthritis the "Nation's Number One Crippler," and states: "There is no permanent cure at present, and even early treatment cannot always forestall severe disability."

With such a gloomy state of affairs prevailing in our country, anyone attempting to speak or write on a subject of such magnitude is assuming a great responsibility. I am well aware of this responsibility, and am willing to assume it because I have spent over fifty years studying this subject in every possible manner. Not only did I witness the ups and downs of arthritis in my wife and countless other patients in my fifty years of practice, but I have also experimented with my own body. Unbelievable as it may sound, my body became so sensitized that I reached the point where I could produce the symptoms of arthritis in a few weeks, and then rid myself of those symptoms in a week or two.

If I felt as pessimistic concerning the chances of arresting arthritis as the majority of doctors feel, I would not dream of writing this book. However, after many years of study, research, and experimenting on my own body, I have come to the definite conclusion that arthritis can be helped, arrested, and prevented in almost all cases—if—and only if—the patient will read carefully and follow the simple and natural plan I am about to place before you.

The task of putting down the results of fifty years of work in a volume of this size is not an easy one, but I will do my best. In return I will ask you to read and re-read every word carefully. Ponder my words, and then do your best to follow my simple plan. It is a plan which I have tested and re-tested many times in numerous cases of arthritis as well as on my own body.

There are too many sick people in our country. Sick people make a sick nation. That may be one of the reasons why the news in our daily papers is so depressing. My aim is not only to help you to get rid of arthritis, but also make you a healthier person than you have been for a long time.

One goes with the other. A person with arthritis is sick in the joints. (That is why the disease is called arthritis. *Arthros* means "joint," and *"itis"* means "inflammation of".) You can be sure that when the joints are inflamed, other parts of the body are also damaged. So, by ridding yourself of arthritis you will benefit your entire body at the same time. The job before you and me is not easy, but it is a most worthwhile one, so let's work together and get on with our project.

First, let me give you a review of my background and the events which led me into a specialized study of arthritis. After that we will go into the day-by-day detailed plan of combating arthritis, and finally I will set down a few suggestions on how you can regain optimum health of your entire body.

Some people live in parts of the country where many of the fruits and vegetables are not available in the winter, or are too expensive, when available. In such cases it is *very important* to resort to *sprouted seeds*. Sprouts furnish an excellent source of natural nutrition; they are very rich in vitamins and minerals.

In addition, sprouts are easy to produce and cost very little. For this reason, we have devoted a chapter to the preparation and use of sprouts. Please read this chapter carefully. It is very important, as it shows you how to add green, *living* food to your diet plan.

Philip J. Welsh, D.D.S., N.D.

MORE ABOUT DR. WELSH

This health manual tells the true story of how Philip J. Welsh, D.D.S., N.D., developed a drugless, nutrition-oriented plan for combating arthritis. He proved this method to be totally effective back in 1923, and was the first person to evolve the method. During his 50 years of practice as a dentist, he gave his patients nutritional counseling and helped thousands of them with their arthritis problems. His research in the field of nutrition, especially concerning arthritis, is of world-wide importance, but has yet to be recognized.

Dr. Welsh's professional career began with a pre-medical course at New York University. He then entered the New York College of Dentistry, graduating in 1917. He gave a series of lectures at The American School of Naturopathy in New York City, which was headed by the famous Benedict Lust, N.D., M.D. Dr. Welsh received the degree of N.D. (Doctor of Naturopathy) in 1926 from this college.

In 1929, he wrote a course entitled *The Seven Essentials of Health*, which was sold nationally and internationally. He received many letters attesting to the efficacy of the plan outlined in the course, which was possibly the first work on holistic health and healing in our century, after several pioneers worked in this field in the 1800's. Dr. Welsh *lived* the truths in the course before he wrote it, and *lived* them for the remainder of his life.

Why is it that this great discovery is not more generally known, even among nutritionists? It is because one must *live* these experiences, as Dr. Welsh did, and also engage in *constant experimentation on one's own body*, not in a laboratory. It is because the great truth "we are what we eat" has not penetrated the medical establishment, which continues to look in the wrong direction for health — to drugs.

Dr. Welsh spent a lifetime helping others find health. His practical experience with arthritis was so extensive — over fifty years — and his method of combating it so unique and effective, that he and I — his partner for fifteen years — decided to write this book — for the present and future generations.

Bianca Leonardo, N.D.

(Clayton School of Natural Healing, Birmingham, Alabama)

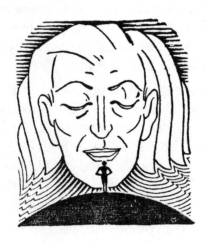

Mind is the Master power that moulds and makes,
And Man is Mind, and evermore he takes
The seal of Thought, and shaping what he wills,
Brings forth a thousands joys, a thousand ills—
He thinks in secret, and it comes to pass:
Environment is but his looking-glass.

FOREWORD

The volume in your hand, and the tremendously important information it contains, is a milestone in health history. You are fortunate to be reading it.

Dr. Welsh's great discovery is yet to be recognized by the establishment, which is making little progress out of the "Dark Ages" of medicine. In the prevailing mode of medicine, germs and viruses are considered to be the principal causes of diseases, rather than poor nutrition and health-hurting habits and lifestyles; drugs and surgery are considered almost the sole solutions to health problems. We have a long way to go to become truly civilized in our style of medicine, the original meaning of the word being: "the healing art."

In our time, "medicine" has become "big business." Prevention is not profitable, nor is nutritional counseling. A great discovery, like the one in this book, is ignored by the establishment. Dr. Philip J. Welsh could only give his message via a book, and reach people one by one with it.

This health manual contains a wealth of vision, common sense, and practical information that is priceless. For someone who is in constant pain with arthritis, who cannot work or enjoy life, such information would be cheap at $1,000. Truly, no price can be put on a message like this. And it works. Dr. Welsh proved it, in his own lifetime, first with his wife, then with his friends and patients, throughout a 50-year career as a dentist. He included his advanced nutritional counseling, and shared his vast experience with health and disease, and especially the arthritic condition, free of charge. So he expressed love for mankind.

For many years, Dr. Welsh pointed out that our national medical agencies and the medical profession as a whole have been and are emphatically stating that *nutrition has **nothing** to do with arthritis.*

He also stated, for he knew beyond a shadow of a doubt, that *nutrition has everything to do with arthritis.*

The experimental method — of giving arthritis patients one food at a time and watching reactions (the mono-diet) — is ORIGINAL WITH DR. WELSH. He devised this experimental method many years ago, when *he healed his wife of rheumatoid arthritis in 1923.* The details are in this manual, in Chapter II. It tells the true story of how Dr. Welsh *developed a drugless, nutrition-oriented plan for combating arthritis in 1923!*

The negative reaction to certain foods is called allergy by many medical practitioners. Dr. Welsh, with his over-half-a-century experience, knows this is not the case. It is simpler than that.

His health-restoring and life-saving message is this: Natural foods agree with the body; unnatural, processed foods and non-foods are toxic to the body, resulting in pain and disease.

This health manual contains a revolutionary, yet simple, *plan that works.* By publishing this sixth edition, the authors are benefactors to humanity.

And now, read, enjoy, utilize, practice and share the treasure that is in your hands: FREEDOM FROM ARTHRITIS THROUGH NUTRITION, a Guidebook for Pain-Free Living.

/s/ Robert S. Mendelsohn, M.D.

(Author of: *Confessions of a Medical Heretic; Malepractice: How Doctors Manipulate Women,* and *How to Have a Healthy Child in Spite of Your Doctor.)*

CONTENTS

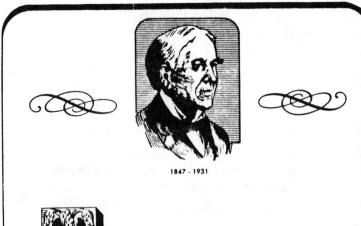

1847 - 1931

The doctor of the future
will give no medicine
but will interest his patients
in the care of the human frame,
in diet, and in the cause and
prevention of disease.

Thomas A. Edison

Note: Since Edison's day, this has begun to happen. It is called "Holistic Medicine." The three words, *whole, holy* and *health* have the same root, and deep thought should be given to how these powerful words are related.

The *whole person* must be treated—body, mind and spirit. Man is not mere matter, to be treated with material substances (especially drugs). He is also mind and spirit; hope, faith, positive thinking, prayer, and natural living, need to be integral parts of his life, for true health and happiness.

Bianca Leonardo, N. D.

CHAPTER I

THE ORIGIN OF MY RESEARCH

Throughout the entire duration of both my pre-medical and dental courses of study, the subject of nutrition was not only neglected but completely overlooked. Not a single reference was made to this very important subject in any of the courses that were offered. As a result, the members of the healing professions were severely lacking in knowledge of the principles of proper nutrition.

All attention was, and still is, focused on the germ theory as the cause of disease. The cures for the germs supposedly producing diseases were and are drugs and medicines. When the patient gets well, drugs take the credit; when the patient dies, God takes the blame.

After my first three years of practicing dentistry in confined quarters, with little exercise and an improper diet, I was stricken with a severe lung condition. Several doctors were engaged to cure me. Various medicines were prescribed; none helped. Instead, my condition worsened, and finally developed into a very serious case of double pneumonia. When things looked darkest, something remarkable happened—I lost my desire for all foods excepting citrus fruits, and for them I had a strong craving. After a few days on this limited diet of citrus, the improvement in my condition was dramatic!

This made a deep impression on me, and it was then, in 1920, that my interest was aroused in the importance of nutrition. I read everything I could get hold of on the subject. The more I learned and put into practice, the more my condition improved, until finally I became well. My interest in nutrition grew. I decided to specialize in nutrition and preventive dentistry. Soon I was lecturing on the subject of *Preventive Dentistry Through Nutrition* to the children in the public schools of New York City, under the auspices of the New York Tuberculosis Association.

In 1925, the Chicago Dental Society embarked on a public service project in the form of an Oral Hygiene Week. During that week talks were to be given over the radio on oral hygiene and tooth decay prevention. To secure material for these radio talks, the Chicago Dental Society announced a contest open to all dentists in the United States to submit twenty-minute essays on the subject of oral hygiene.

Now, at that time — the early '20's — the prevailing and well-established theory was — "A clean tooth never decays." Through my practice of preventive dentistry and original research, I found that this theory was *not true.* I found that even though patients kept their teeth scrupulously clean, their teeth continued to decay if their diet included refined sugar and was lacking in valuable nutrients.

In the essay that I submitted to the Chicago Dental Society, I pointed out this *revolutionary finding — that adequate nutrition is most essential for preventing tooth decay.*

In December of that year, the judging committee of the Chicago Dental Society sent me a letter announcing that I was chosen a winner in this contest — one of seven winners. The letter is reproduced on the next page.

I was the first dentist in the nation to advocate proper nutrition for the prevention of tooth decay.

What has all this to do with arthritis? You will soon learn.

CHICAGO DENTAL SOCIETY

December 3, 1925

Dr. Philip Welsh
37 West 57th St.
New York, New York

Dear Dr. Welsh:

The Public Service Committee of the Chicago
Dental Society takes great pleasure in announcing
to you that you have been successful in winning
one of the seven $50.00 prizes offered for the best
twenty-minute speech suitable for a radio audience.

There was much excellent material received,
and it required a great deal of effort to determine
the winners. Because of this keen competition, you
are to be especially congratulated for your splendid
essay.

You will find enclosed our check for $50.00,
which is indeed a small compensation for the valuable
service you have rendered this committee. We wish
to thank you most heartily for your cooperation.

Yours very truly,

F. Blaine Rhobotham

For
PUBLIC SERVICE COMMITTEE

CHAPTER II

HOW GRACE WELSH CONQUERED ARTHRITIS

In the summer of 1923, my wife was stricken with a severe case of rheumatoid arthritis. She was in constant pain, day and night. She could not sleep, turn in bed, or hardly move at all without severe pain. The doctor prescribed medicines, but instead of improving, her condition became worse. So we decided to discontinue the drugs and resort to nutrition and natural methods. Here are the exact steps that were taken:

THE CLEANSING PROCESS

To give Nature a chance to heal the body, we instituted an internal cleansing routine. The bowels were cleared with a lukewarm enema every morning and evening for one week.

One of the main causes of arthritis is an accumulation of toxic matter in various parts of the body. The only way to get permanent relief is to rid the body of these toxic wastes.

The enema is a simple, harmless and most effective way of cleansing the body of some of these waste products. Many people, especially those on in years, have sluggish bowels, and as a result, they carry an internal cesspool in their bodies. These putrefactive wastes permeate the system, causing a great many ailments. To counteract this disease-producing condition, the enema, properly used, is of tremendous value. I want to stress the words *properly used*. Most people do not know the right method, so please follow the method outlined here.

THE PROPER WAY TO TAKE AN ENEMA

1. If you do not have one, purchase a two-quart rubber enema bag. (Do not get a hot water bottle, which is a different item.)

18

2. Completely fill it with lukewarm water and suspend from a height of about six feet. (Use shower door or a nail, etc.)

3. To facilitate the hanging, take a piece of wire and shape it like an "S." This will help you hang the enema bag.

4. Lubricate both the nozzle and anus (rectal opening) with vaseline.

5. Expel the air from the tube by letting some of the water to escape through the nozzle. Then close the clamp.

6. Carefully insert the nozzle into the rectum.

7. Open the control clamp and allow about half of the water in the bag to slowly flow into the lower bowels.

8. Compress the clamp to stop the flow of water and remove the nozzle.

9. Give the water and fecal matter time to be expelled.

10. Completely fill the bag again and repeat the process, but this time allow about 3/4 of the water in the bag to flow into the bowels.

11. Remove the nozzle and allow the bowels to empty.

12. Repeat the process, but this time allow the entire contents of the bag to flow into the bowels. If at any time you feel too much pressure, stop the flow of water by compressing the clamp, and wait a few minutes; then complete the process.

13. After the bowels have completely emptied, wash the parts with soap and COLD water; then dry the parts.

If you have never taken an enema, all this may seem quite involved, but after a short while you will find it simple and beneficial. If you find it difficult or inconvenient to use the enema, you can instead, have a series of *colonics*. With this method, a machine is used which sends water into the bowels and intestines, and cleans out all waste matter that is lodged in the body and never is released with ordinary bowel movements. Colonics are given by practitioners who specialize in this practice; many chiropractors offer this service. If you would like to hasten the healing process, you can do so by *fasting* a day or two, simultaneously with the cleansing process — before starting the new diet. (See further details on *fasting* in Chapter 4.)

COLEMICS FOR INTESTINAL CLEANSING

There is yet a third way to accomplish colon cleansing—the colemic (pronounced ko-lē'-mik). One may say that the colemic is a method between the enema and the colonic technique. One purchases equipment for his own bathroom, a so-called "colemic board."

Sea Klenz Intestinal Cleansers

The digestive tract is as much a lifeline of the body as the bloodstream. Today, the average diet is filled with chemicals and preservatives, over-processed foods and a lack of fiber.

Wachters' Sea Klenz Intestinal Cleansers are specifically formulated to counteract some of these harmful effects, and will help promote proper digestion and elimination, remove stagnation and maintain daily colon health. They are all natural, non-habit forming, bulk fiber cleansers, whose main ingredient is organic sea vegetation.

Sea Klenz is non-abrasive, soothing, and is used for: (1) constipation, or to prevent same; (2) malabsorption; and (3) a preparation for the colonic regime.

The ingredients of the original formula (called 51-B) are: A combination of Sodium Alginate from sea vegetation; Psyllium seed husks; dehydrated lemon powder; cereal solids, and a Wachters' blend of sea plants. Sea Klenz is not found in stores.

Call 800-350-LIFE for a source.

Pre-Colemic Information

The small intestine is the area where most food absorption occurs. Its parts are: the duodenum and the anterior portion, including the jejunum and the ileum.

The main function of the large intestine is the absorption of water. It consists of these parts: the cecum, the ascending colon, the transverse colon, the descending colon, the sigmoid colon, the rectum, and the anal canal—forming a kind of frame around the abdominal cavity. (See diagram in Appendix; also charts depicting colon conditions.)

In preparing for a colemic, no food should be consumed for at least ten hours. Upon awakening, or at least three hours before the colemic, Wachters' Sea Klenz should be taken.

The purpose in taking an intestinal cleanser prior to a colemic is that the colemic empties the large intestine of wastes, bacteria, etc., but not the small intestine. Sea Klenz helps to push (like a broom) fecal material and wastes from the small intestine, where the colemic does not act.

Herbal Fiber #750 and #751 by Enzymatic Therapy also contain ingredients that help rid the body of parasites and yeast overgrowth. (Ask your health food store.)

The colemic cleansing process is a gradual one, and after the bowels are cleansed, the water loosens caked-up residues on the inside lining. The bacteria, mucus-ridden excrement is expelled into the toilet, where it belongs! Patience is necessary, because the body is not always ready to release its poisons all at once.

You must be willing to do this — in order to heal your body!

There are many positive effects from colon cleansing. One is that the lymphatics become unblocked, appetite is regained, absorption is greatly increased, mental abilities are improved, the eyes clear, one can work longer hours without fatigue, the disposition improves. (Toxins make one irritable, angry, sluggish, mean!)

And, of course, toxins make one sick.   It is truly said that "death begins in the colon."

The people of the world are polluted within — and this causes antagonisms and strife — because the internal toxins make people angry, as well as sick.

This is so important that we wish to emphasize it: **Colonics and Colemics not only cleanse the body but the mind!** When the body is loaded with toxins (and everyone's is — unless they are cleaning the colon frequently) — the person becomes irritable and angry — the toxins affect the mind.

Contrariwise, after a colon cleansing, one becomes kind, amiable, loving — as well as getting a big surge of energy.

We must not only eat properly but assimilate and eliminate.

Mere emptying the bowels on the toilet is not enough. You have a choice of a *Colemic* (at home — you do the process yourself, or with the help of a family member)— or a *Colonic* (where you go to the office of a health practitioner who gives colonics).

Just one of either will not do the job!   The first few times you have the colonic or colemic (the latter is more thorough) — you will notice that the process helps soften and carry away intestinal debris. But the real cleansing comes after this intestinal putrefaction is removed, and one actually gets down to the mucus in the lining of the intestines.

Research has demonstrated that the colon has reflex points that affect the organs — so the physical process of the water entering and being expelled has a toning effect — not only on the intestinal system, but also on stimulating the various organs.

A well-developed tissue cleansing system is very good to help overcome pain in all parts of the body.

In working to overcome a serious degenerative disease, it is recommended that the treatment be ongoing and constantly applied. Every other day is best, for the first week. If the patient drops in energy suddenly, the process must be halted.

It should be understood that this treatment is not a cure-all, but an important step in the detoxification program.

This detoxification program is very powerful. Tremendous healing can be accomplished!

Not all the toxins are expelled. Some of them go back into the system. Therefore, if it is at all possible, go into a wet sauna — the same or the next day. Those toxins which are in the circulatory system are pushed out through the skin.

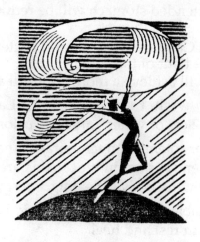

"Nothing in Nature is unbeautiful."
—Lord Alfred Tennyson

Benefits of Colonics and
Colemics

After a colonic or colemic, (or series of them), you can expect:

(1) Your eyes to lighten in color;

(2) Sores on the body to heal more quickly;

(3) Increased energy;

(4) Clearer thinking;

(5) A general feeling of well-being;

(6) The skin will glow with radiance;

(7) Joint and back pain will lessen;

(8) Darker skin on the genitals and rectum will lighten (the dark flesh indicates blood stagnation);

(9) The appetite will increase;

(10) An extended stomach will be reduced, with repeated treatments;

(11) Much Candida Albicans and bacteria will be washed out of the colon;

(12) You will achieve a more youthful appearance.

You may wish to use Bacillus Laterosporous (2 tablespoons in 2 oz. of water), after the colonic/colemic.

A colonic or colemic can temporarily make you feel weak because a tremendous amount of toxins are eliminated from the body. When the body is healing, energy is consumed.

It is advisable to take your colemic before retiring, so that the body can rest and heal.

Instructions for the Colemic

Upon receiving your colemic board, assemble according to instructions. Purchase a five-gallon plastic bucket with a handle.

The colemic board can be positioned at any angle, so it fits in virtually any bathroom. The part of the board with the catheter rests on the toilet seat, and the back of the board rests on a chair or the bathtub.

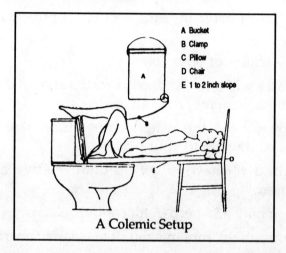

A Bucket
B Clamp
C Pillow
D Chair
E 1 to 2 inch slope

A Colemic Setup

Wash the bucket with hydrogen peroxide or bleach. Get it super clean. The bucket must be at least three feet above the board. It can be placed on a table, wooden box or crate or improvised in some way. It could be suspended from a hook in the ceiling. Half fill the bucket before suspending it. Use water as warm as possible, but watch the temperature. If the water is hot to your hand, it will be hotter to the rectum. Warm water expands the intestine, and allows for much more rapid expulsion of toxic wastes.

Filling the hose: First, clamp the hose. One end of the hose has a plastic "L"; turn the hose upside down. This part has a metal weight in it. You are going to start pouring water into the rubber tube. As soon as one section is filled, unclamp and pour more water in; then reclamp. In other words, the entire tube has to be totally filled with water. The air must be out of the tube. It works by reverse gravity. It is called siphoning.

The next step: fill the bucket to top, using another container to do so. Then put thumb over top of rubber tube (you don't want any air to get in or water to get out), and invert it, place the weighted tube into the bucket. It will go right down to the bottom.

Insert the catheter into the rectum approximately two inches.

You are ready for your colemic!

The water will enter and exit with fecal matter from the rectum. The advantages over an enema are:

(1) You control the water temperature. You can add more hot or cold water to your bucket;

(2) You don't have to get up until the five gallons of water are used;

(3) You may add herbs, chlorophyll, etc.;

(4) You can do implants with the colemic board;

(5) You can change your position: you can sit up, you can lie down, you can turn to your right side or left side; you can have your knees up and bent, or legs straight.

(6) As the water enters, you can release it at any time by pushing out. You can allow the water to go further by taking a deep breath and expanding your abdomen; permit the water to go up as far as you desire. If there is too much pressure, there is fecal blockage.

(7) The intestine has pockets called villi (finger-like projections), where these toxins and poisons are trapped, so don't expect it to happen all at once. You will have a major breakthrough! You can't expect to do just one intestinal cleaning.

(8) You can massage different parts of your body; this triggers the release of the fecal matter. Your thumb or finger can be placed on a hard mass, which will start pulsating and trigger a release. Then you might exclaim: "Oh, what a feeling!"

(9) Letting go of fecal matter, toxins, and poisons physically can also simultaneously release *mental* poisons and toxins. This release is a total catharsis.

(10)   While this is going on, you can declare, mentally or audibly: "I am letting go of old things in my life I no longer need; they no longer belong there. I feel strong. I have no fear. I am clean!"

Implants

Implants should not be attempted with a dirty colon, because you will reabsorb the toxins. After some intestinal cleaning, perhaps three weeks, implantation can be attempted.

Another name for implants is rectal feeding. Nutrients are absorbed very readily through the rectum. Rectal feeding differs from a colonic in that nutritional liquids are implanted into the rectum, and held for 5-15 minutes. Substances that can be used: herbs, garlic (macerate and add to water); herbal teas; chlorophyll (liquid chlorophyll is available in food stores).

One rule: never irritate the mucous membrane. The substances should be soothing, healing, not irritating. Don't make the solutions too strong. H_2O_2 (hydrogen peroxide) should only be attempted under the supervision of a health professional.

Bacillus Laterosporus liquid may be used as an implant after several colemics. See page 99 for more information on this product.

Notes: The material on these pages first appeared in Tree of Life's book: *A Holistic Protocol for the Immune System*, by Scott J. Gregory, O. M. D.

Information on a source for the colemic board is available by calling or writing this publisher.

THE DIET CONTROL PROGRAM

After the bowel cleansing routine is completed, the next step is Diet Control. *What one eats will depend upon the time of year and the foods available.*

Grace was stricken in the summertime, when the *sweet seedless grapes* were in season and in plentiful supply. She ate them *exclusively* for the first four days. The results were dramatic. Most of her pain disappeared! She was able to move and walk without pain.

On the fifth day, *sweet, ripe watermelon* was added to her diet. *She was permitted to eat all she desired of these two foods* and she felt *satisfied.* Her body was being *cleansed* by these *cleansing fruits.* Pleased with the lessening of pain, she did not find it difficult to adhere to this strict regime of diet.

After one week on the seedless grapes and watermelon diet, fresh corn on the cob was added. Young ears were chosen, and these were prepared with a minimum of cooking. You will find in Chapter VIII our method for the proper preparation of sweet corn. Fresh corn is very nourishing; it is packed with vitamins and minerals. Really, one is eating seed kernels, each with the potential of becoming a plant itself; that is why each kernel is packed with nutrition power! We consider sweet corn to be "the king of vegetables." Grace ate the corn alone, without adding salt or salty butter. Why these must not be used will be explained later.

MY ORIGINAL, EXPERIMENTAL METHOD

These three foods: sweet, seedless grapes, sweet, ripe watermelon, and fresh corn on the cob were our basic foods. They were used for one week, to make sure they were compatible (agreeable). BY ADDING ONE FOOD AT A TIME, we were able to screen each item to find out if that food was suitable or not for Grace's condition. *This experimental method is the simplest and surest way to develop a diet for one troubled with arthritis — and other diseases!*

If too many foods are added at one time, and pain or other symptoms of arthritis, such as redness, swelling, etc., return, then we do not know which of the foods is to blame. But by adding one food at a time and using it steadily for one week, we can then immediately tell whether that food is beneficial or not — and if not, eliminate it from the diet at once. This experimental method, which I originated, *really works!*

NOTE: I wish to strongly emphasize here that these three foods are not the only ones that may be used to begin perfecting the proper diet. *Any fruit that is in season* and available may be used. During the winter months many areas of our country have a very limited supply of fresh fruits. In such cases, use whatever is available.

Apples, being a year-round fruit, may be the only fruit available in your location. In this case, use apples only, as a mono-diet for several days, until the arthritis pain lessens. Be sure to peel the apples, in order to avoid the residue of chemical sprays that are being used on our foods. If you can procure organic fruit, you are fortunate.

After that, *add any fruit or vegetable, only one at a time,* and watch the reaction on your body. If it agrees with you and does not cause any pain, then add that food to your list of basic foods.

If you cannot obtain any fresh fruit or fresh vegetables you may be obliged to resort to frozen foods. If you must use frozen foods, read the labels to make sure they do not contain salt or other chemicals as flavorings or preservatives.

Fruits (raw, uncooked) are cleansing foods. *Do not use canned fruits.* The important point I want you to grasp is that wherever you live, you should not give up trying to help yourself get rid of arthritis because you are unable to obtain the good supply of natural foods that people in California and Florida are blessed with.

THE BASIC CLEANSING FRUITS

The following *fresh fruits* not only nourish the body, but also cleanse the intestinal tract. They should be ripe.

Avocados and bananas are excellent, natural foods, but are not in the cleansing fruit category. They may be used later.

Apples	Mangoes	Pears
Apricots	Melons: Cantaloupe,	Persimmons
Cherries	Casaba, Crenshaw	Pineapple
Figs	Honeydew, Watermelon	Plums (sweet)
Grapes	Nectarines	Sapotas
Loquats	Peaches	

All these fruits are basic cleansing fruits. After being on any of these cleansing fruits for a week or two, you may add:

Oranges	Grapefruits	Lemons
Tomatoes	Strawberries and other Berries	

The latter group should be added cautiously, for most of these fruits are picked before they are ripe, and, as a result, may create a problem. So, in adding any of the above fruits, make sure they are ripe and pleasant to the taste.

GRACE'S RECOVERY

By adhering to the aforementioned list of natural foods, and the others described in Chapter IV, my wife not only got rid of arthritis, but regained her over-all health and energy and lived to a ripe old age, active to the end. She did not remain on such a restricted diet, but afterwards was careful in her eating. She gave up her habit of daily pies and cakes with coffee and sugar.

One cannot eat everything "in sight," ingest many harmful substances, and expect to be free from arthritis and other diseases! When any processed foods are eaten, Nature rebels in the form of pain and disease. This should be remembered, in order to have a life free from suffering.

TEMPORARY RELIEF OF ARTHRITIS PAIN

Pain is Nature's warning that the body is being abused in one way or another. If we can determine in what way we are causing this abuse and then stop it, the body then heals itself, and the pain stops. This may take a few days or a few weeks. In the meantime, we can obtain *temporary* relief by massaging the parts that hurt (or getting a professional massage) and then applying heat in any one of the following ways:

1. Exposing the part to sunshine.

2. Applying a hot water bottle to the aching part. If you do not have a hot water bottle, you can use any bottle that has a screw cap, fill it with very hot water, then wrap it in a towel held in place with one or two elastic bands or a string.

3. Apply an electric heating pad to the aching part.

4. Apply a towel dipped in hot water; wring out.

5. Immerse the aching part in hot water.

Arthritis pain is worse during the night, especially during cold weather. Heat, as directed above, will give you temporary relief.

CHAPTER III

WHAT CAUSES ARTHRITIS?

Three of the main causes are what we call the "THREE BAD WHITES":

WHITE SUGAR   WHITE FLOUR   SALT

This should never be forgotten by one who is troubled by arthritis.

Unfortunately, these three harmful substances are very common in the American diet.

"But what can I use in their place?" you will immediately ask.

SUBSTITUTES FOR SUGAR

Use *Honey, Pure Maple Syrup*, Pure Maple Sugar*, or Blackstrap Molasses* in your beverages, on cereals, etc., where you ordinarily use white sugar; also in candies or baked confections.

*We understand that these products are expensive. But if you do use maple syrup, be sure it is *pure* Vermont syrup, and not mixed with sugar, as the lower grade often is. This is true of maple sugar also — be sure it is pure and not mixed with white sugar.

Entire books have been written on the extreme harmfulness of sugar and you should read at least one.

Most of all, remember that the body does not need all those sweets the average American pours into it. Nature gives us natural sweets in dates, raisins, other dried fruits, fresh fruits, nuts, seeds, and honey. These are good for us (in moderation) but the processed white sugar and the confections made from it, are extremely harmful.

SUBSTITUTE FOR WHITE FLOUR

Use whole grain flour instead of white flour. As you advance with the natural diet, you will find less desire for breads and pastries.

SUBSTITUTES FOR SALT

No. 1

Here is a good salt substitute: Combine powdered kelp, garlic powder, mild chili powder, and Brewer's Yeast powder (available at health food stores.) Put the mixture into your salt shaker and use it in place of salt. If the shaker has large holes, it will shake like salt.

You should use one teaspoon of the other items to 1/2 cup of Brewer's Yeast. These proportions may be varied to suit your taste. There are many types of Brewer's Yeast; each has its own flavor.

Also, cultivate the use of natural herbs for seasoning. Herb charts and books are available at health food stores and some bookstores. Two good herbs are dill weed and mild chili powder. Use the latter sparingly. Onion and garlic will also take the place of salt.

Check out what products are available in your local health food store. Two multi-purpose liquids that taste salty but contain no salt, are: Bragg Liquid Aminos (from soybeans) and Dr. Bernard Jensen's Quick-Sip (plant products only). Both can be used as bouillon bases for soups and as seasonings.

At first you will miss the salt, but as time goes on, your taste buds will change, and you will learn to enjoy the natural flavors of the various foods. Then you will not require so much seasoning.

In all cases of arthritis, high blood pressure, overweight and for health in general, it is important to avoid the use of salt.

SALT SUBSTITUTE NO. 2

1 cup of Brewer's Yeast

2 teaspoons of powdered kelp

1 teaspoon of mild chili pepper

1 or 2 cloves of minced garlic

The proportions may be varied to suit your taste.

WHY NOT SALT?

Years ago, famed French surgeon Dr. Jean Bouchom penned a medical report calling salt the most injurious of modern food poisons. "It is damaging to both body and mind," he wrote, "and it should be banished."

Jethro Kloss wrote: "Common salt contains chloride of sodium, which is an inorganic mineral and cannot be used by any cell structure of the body. It irritates the stomach and bloodstream, is indigestible, and hinders the digestion of other foods. It is one of the causes of rheumatism, dizziness, cancer and scurvy; it puts harmful minerals into the system."

Otto Carqué, in *Vital Facts About Foods*, wrote: "The salt eating habit may be acquired as any other unhygienic habit, but if we choose our foods rightly, there is absolutely no necessity for it."

After our foods are broken down by the process of digestion, the resulting nutrients enter the individual cells by osmosis through the cell wall or membrane. By the same process the cells dispose of their waste products. The process is known as metabolism.

This important interchange of nutrients and waste products through the cell depends upon the concentration of sodium in the blood. Just as soon as the concentration of sodium is increased through the use of salt, this very important function of the body cells is interfered with, causing death of the cells — which ultimately brings on many ailments.

This conclusion has been well established by many researchers. That is why doctors who realize the importance of proper nutrition are recommending a low sodium or salt-free diet in cases of migraine, epilepsy, insomnia, nervous tension, dropsy, and *especially* in cases of high blood pressure, and obesity. I would add *Arthritis,* for in my over 50 years of experience with arthritis, I have found that as long as the patient continues to use any salt or any salted foods, it is impossible to get rid of arthritis. That is the reason I strongly recommend that those who are troubled with arthritis should strictly avoid the use of any food that has been seasoned with salt — and that includes so-called "sea-salt."

Commercial salt substitutes are not advised either, as they contain some salt, and chemicals that aggravate arthritic conditions.

The use of salt is also a factor in causing high blood pressure. Those who have arthritis are, as a rule, excessive salt-eaters, and naturally when they give up salt, they miss it. However, each day that they do without salt, their yearning for it lessens and believe it or not, when they go back and try to use salt indiscriminately the way they formerly did, they find it objectionable.

A powerful indictment of salt, entitled *Killer Salt,* appeared in 1977. The author, Marietta Whittlesey, wrote it out of her own life experience, plus much research. Unfortunately, the book is now out of print.

HERBS FOR SEASONING

In a health food store or bookstore, you should get a book on the use of herbs. It will help you greatly in making your foods tasty, and as a result, you will not miss the salt. There are a number of healthful seasonings available today in health food stores. Read the list of ingredients, to be sure salt is not one of them.

WHY NOT SUGAR?

"Refined sugar has justly earned for itself the name of 'Calcium or Lime Thief.' The natural sugar in the sugar cane has a large proportion of calcium combined with it. In the refining process, this important mineral is extracted and lost. The refined sugar is now sucrose, and because of its natural affinity for calcium, it unites with the calcium present in the digestive tract and in the bloodstream. *Calcium saccarate*, the new substance formed, is thrown off because it cannot be retained and used in the blood, thereby robbing the system of the calcium which was originally present in it. *Calcium* is needed for building and maintaining sound bones and teeth, and clotting of the blood.

"The use of refined or unnatural sugar is therefore more injurious than most persons realize, and it is better to eat natural sweets — in the form of dates, sweet fruits and honey. One may eat all the fruits he or she wishes. However, dates and honey are concentrated, and should be used in moderation. In recipes, use half to two-thirds the amount of honey that is called for in sugar. It is simple to eliminate the 'three bad whites' and make wholesome substitutions. But the less cooking of food the better. Use more salads, fresh fruits and other uncooked foods.

"*After many tests, I found that as long as the patient continued to use refined sugar, it was impossible to get rid of arthritis.*" (From *The Seven Essentials of Health*, Philip J. Welsh, first published in 1929.)

As stated earlier, I was the first dentist in the nation to state that sugar was harmful to the teeth. Now it is common knowledge, but few persons care enough about avoiding tooth decay, to eliminate sugar from their diet. The choice is yours!

After my work, *The Seven Essentials of Health* appeared, other books came out, with even stronger statements against sugar. However, the use of refined sugar is so widespread, with the amount being used greatly increasing every year, that most persons assume there is nothing wrong with it.

But the opposite is true! A large number of researchers have studied the effects of sugar on the human body and have definitely proven that it is a dangerous product.

Dr. John Yudkin, M.D., calls it "The Quiet Killer" that can cause heart disease, diabetes, ulcers and other often-fatal diseases. This distinguished scientist reveals startling new facts about sugar in his book *Sweet and Dangerous*, a headline-making book. He says that the ordinary table sugar you eat every day can kill you, and explains, clearly and concisely, why this sugar is a crucial health hazard for all ages — in fact, is deadly dangerous. Dr. Yudkin, a renowned physician, biochemist and researcher, was professor of Physiology, Nutrition and Dietetics at Queen Elizabeth College of London University. He writes:

". . . My research on coronary disease has convinced me beyond doubt that sugar plays a considerable part in this terrifying modern epidemic . . . . If only a fraction of what is already known about the effects of sugar were to be revealed, the use of that substance would promptly be banned."

Dr. Yudkin has done a noble deed in writing this book, and it should be read widely.

In his booklet, *Sugar, the Curse of Civilization*, J.I. Rodale wrote: "The practice of eating refined sugar deprives the body of essential vitamins and minerals . . . Sugar robs the body of its Vitamin B, called Thiamine, which is destroyed. Thiamine is one of the most important vitamins for good health. It is necessary for growth, good appetite, and smooth functioning of the digestive tract. It plays so big a part in nerve health that it is called the 'morale' vitamin. Most important of all, Thiamine is vitally concerned with the digestion and assimilation of all carbohydrate foods — the sugars and starches. It must be present in considerable quantity if these foods are to be used at all by the body."

In another book, *Natural Health, Sugar and the Criminal Mind*, the same author, founder of *Prevention* magazine, presents a powerful indictment of sugar in what it does to the mind. Many criminals (including Hitler) were and are sugar addicts, as sugar adversely affects the bloodstream, and then the brain.

Carleton Wade wrote an article: *"How Nutrition May Tame Violence,"* (Let's Live magazine, August 1972). This famous nutritionist gives case histories of retarded, hyperactive, troublesome, fighting, uncontrollable, unteachable children, who consumed many sugary sweets. When their diet was changed, they became "as good as gold." He also has evidence on criminals who were sugar addicts. The sugar causes neurological disorders which predispose the instinct to kill.

Sugar Blues, a book by William Dufty, was published in 1975. The author was an obese sugar addict until he managed to kick the habit; he became a slender, handsome, vigorous anti-sugar campaigner. The book gives the entire history of sugar and is a real eye opener. Dufty writes:

"Sugar is a national plague; it is slow poison to millions of people. To other millions it means instant stress. Virtually an entire nation is pre-diabetic by diagnostic standards. Worldwide scientific research now links sugar with multiple major diseases . . . . Yet we have become captive customers of sugar-pushing (interests). Food, drinks, cigarettes — all are laced with this hidden poison. How did a great civilization ever slide into such a stupefying bind?"

Dufty quotes many researchers. One states: "Inquiry into the dietary history of patients diagnosed as schizophrenic reveals that the diet of their choice is rich in sweets, candy, cakes, coffee, caffeinated beverages, and foods prepared with sugar. These foods, which stimulate the adrenals, should be eliminated or severely restricted."

He also covers the diseases of diabetics and hypoglycemia, and reveals the relationship of sugar to them.

This book should be required reading by every teacher, parent, and most importantly, by every young person.

Back to Eden, a remarkable book by Jethro Kloss, is called "the classical guide to herbal medicine, natural foods and home remedies." The author states: "Refined white sugar drains out all the mineral salts of the blood, bones and tissues."

Now, you may be wondering about substituting saccharin for sugar. Sorry, that is another poison! W.B. Taylor, Ph.D., who has done research on saccharin, reveals that it is a coal-tar derivative. And what does this substance do in the human system? "We know for a fact that cancer can be caused in 100% of all animals where continued irritation is made by coal tar."

Brown sugar is nothing more than white sugar with some molasses added for color and flavor.

RESTAURANT DINING

When we eat in restaurants we encounter the problem of getting foods that are free from "the three bad whites" — salt, white sugar, and white flour products. One has no control over the ingredients and food products used in restaurants. It is therefore advisable for the arthritis patient to eat at home as much as possible (The latest statistics show that 42% of meals in the U.S. are eaten in restaurants or fast-food eateries. This is an unfortunate trend).

ARTIFICIAL ADDITIVES

In addition to these *three villains,* we must not overlook the many *preservatives and artificial additives* being used so freely in our food supply. These foreign substances do not belong in the body, and when they enter it they cause many disturbances by upsetting the balance of normal metabolism. So, when you begin this regime, it is very important to make sure you do not allow any of these to enter your body.

After one has developed arthritis, one's body becomes sensitized, and the slightest intake of any extraneous matter will interfere with the recovery.

Practically all canned and packaged foods are treated with or combined with sugar, salt, and/or preservatives. These must be strictly avoided. In a body which has developed arthritis, a small amount of any of the above extraneous substances entering the body will prevent its recovery.

BAKING POWDER

Baking powder is another item that should be eliminated from the arthritic's (and any health seeker's) diet. Jethro Kloss, that tireless researcher, wrote: "Baking powder contains two chemicals: Bicarbonate of soda, and tartaric acid. These two chemicals do not neutralize each other in any way so as to destroy or render them harmless, and there is left in the bread a substance identical with Rochelle Salts sold at the drugstore . . . This has no nutritive value, but retards digestion, and gives the eliminative organs extra work to throw off the poison . . . Our present phosphate beds are exhausted, but phosphate is still needed for the making of pancake flour and manufacture of baking powders.

"Aluminum compounds are used extensively with phosphates in the manufacture of fully one-half of all the baking powders manufactured in the United States. The manual of the Parke-Davis Company, one of the largest pharmaceutical houses in America, states concerning aluminum: 'Powerful astringent (causes animal tissue to contract); rarely used internally.'

"Most baking powders on the market now are real poisons. They eat the lining of the stomach or damage it until congestion and inflammation follow. Soda decreases the pancreatic juices, which are used to digest protein, fats and carbohydrates. More than one hundred million pounds of baking powders are used in the United States every year, and less than one million pounds can be said to be free from dangerous poisons."

REMEMBER THIS:

A single chemical or foreign substance taken into the body can keep arthritis troubling you forever. The following three cases will illustrate this fact:

CASE NUMBER ONE

Jim Berger was a widower in his middle sixties. He was suffering with a severe case of arthritis in his hands. He had been through a great deal of medical treatment, with no permanent relief. He was finally sent to me to have his teeth extracted, with the hope that this would relieve him of arthritis.

After X-raying and examining his teeth, I decided *not* to extract them, because they were in good condition.

I put him on a rather strict basic diet. Being a widower and having had no experience in preparing his own food, he had been eating all his meals in restaurants. It was not easy for him to change his eating habits, but he was ready to do anything to get rid of the constant pain in his hands. After two weeks on the basic diet, he had some relief, but still had pain.

Because I thought he was unknowingly eating something that was not on the basic diet, I instructed him to write down every item of food he ate in one week. He did this and brought the data to me. After careful study, I noticed he had used tomato sauce as a seasoning over his salads. I instructed him to eliminate the tomato sauce and report back in two weeks. The following week he called me and was happy to report that his pain was gone. To make sure we had found the right cause of his pain, I advised him to use tomato sauce again. The pain returned, but left after he stopped its use the second time.

This was a good demonstration of the fact that *one wrong item* of food can interfere with the recovery from arthritis.

CASE NUMBER TWO

Another case during my practice was that of a Mrs. Burns.

A wealthy woman in her forties, she was badly crippled with arthritis in her knees and spine. It was apparent to Mrs. Burns that her husband was tired of having a sick and crippled wife. She sensed that he was losing interest in their marriage and, because she was very much in love with him, she was concerned about their imminent separation.

She had tried unsuccessfully for several years to find relief from arthritis, and finally she went to one of the famous clinics, where she received a thorough examination and treatment at great expense, but no improvement.

Her doctors had sent her home with instructions to have her teeth extracted. When she came to me I found her teeth in very good condition and so refused to remove them. Instead, I suggested the Basic Diet in this manual. In three weeks she was not only free from pain, but had gone back to dancing with her husband, a recreation of which they were both fond. The result was, of course, that Mr. Burns renewed his devotion to his healthy, renewed wife.

All was well until about a month later, when she called to report that she had some pain in her knees. I asked her whether she had made any change in diet. The only change she had made was the addition of cottage cheese. Now, cottage cheese not only has a great deal of salt, but other additives as well. I advised her to stop eating cottage cheese, and in a week she was free from all pain.

It was then that I set out to find a salt-free cheese. The result is the recipe for Home-Made Cheese which you will find in this book.

CASE NUMBER THREE

Lilian Wells writes: "When I first met Dr. Welsh during an interview for employment as a secretary, I was so impressed by his dignity of manner and his robust health at eighty years young, that I knew he had something good going for him. I thought to myself, 'If I get the job, I will make it a point to find out what his secret of success is.'

"He did engage me, and it wasn't long before I was emulating him — especially when I learned that he was intensely involved with the problems of arthritis and obesity — because for several years I had been troubled with arthritic pain in my right shoulder. Also, I weighed 15 pounds 'extra'.

"Before beginning to use Dr. Welsh's diet plan, I had a severe rash on the fingers of my right hand. Shortly after adopting his plan, this rash disappeared. Now when I revert to eating some of my former 'junk' foods, this rash reappears.

"The benefits I derived were discernible from the start. In a matter of several weeks not only had my arthritis disappeared, but many of my unwanted extra pounds had, too! I have just had a physical check-up and my doctor says I'm in great shape. It's wonderful to be free from pain and feel slim and youthful again. I am grateful that I have had the good fortune to meet and learn from Dr. Philip J. Welsh."

(Signed, Lilian Wells)

This demonstrates how the body protects itself and rejects what is not good for it. It also demonstrates how a single food item which is not compatible can keep an adverse condition going. With my plan of adding one food at a time, it is possible for the patient to find out which foods are healthful and which are not.

READ THE LABELS

Here is one way to protect yourself from the additives and other harmful ingredients in prepared foods: Carefully read any labels on foods you are about to purchase in the market. As a rule, the ingredients are in very small print, and hard to read for some people. If this is the case with you, you could carry a small pocket magnifying glass, which can make it easier to read the small print.

Only a minority of America's food shoppers read labels. They do not do so because they do not know what to look for, do not realize how important it is to do so, and because the print is too small.

Now that you are reading this book, you are no longer in that class of the "unknowing." You do know now what you must look for, and to protect your health and that of your family, you should read labels. The first ingredient listed is present in the largest quantity. Sometimes there is no information on the package. This does not mean the product is pure. It may be full of chemicals. It is best to avoid these foods, and prepare your own as much as possible. Use more and more natural foods and fewer prepared foods. Natural foods are cheaper and better for your health.

Scrutinize the ingredients listed on the packages of ice cream. Some have many chemicals; others are more healthful.

DANGERS OF ALUMINUM COOKING UTENSILS

A great many authorities* who have investigated the use of aluminum cooking utensils have found that when foods are cooked in such ware, they combine with the aluminum, forming poisonous compounds which are extremely injurious to the human body. In cases of arthritis, it is extremely important to stop using aluminum cooking utensils; instead, use iron, ovenware glass, enameled ware, or stainless steel.

-----

* Harry Gideon Wells, M.D., Professor of Pathology, University of Chicago, researched this thoroughly and made a statement before a Federal agency; Charles T. Betts, M.D.; Hazel Parcelle, D.C., N.D.; Phirozie Nazir, Ph.D; Jethro Kloss and Carleton Wade, health authors; Dr. Victor C. Vaughan, once dean of the Medical Dept. at the Univ. of Michigan, William Held, M.D., Director of the U.S. Health League, Dr. H.A. McGuigan, who wrote in the British Medical Journal, London. There are many others.

EXPERTS POINT TO EVIDENCE LINKING FATTY DIET TO CANCER

(From the Los Angeles Times, Sept. 2, 1977, by George Alexander, Times Science writer.)

In this article, experts stated that a diet rich in fats is one that can cause cancer of the breast and colon. Dr. Adrianne E. Rogers, a physician with the Massachusetts Institute of Technology's Department of Nutrition and Food Science, stated that: "Evidence to support the above contention is accumulating at such a rapid rate that the prudent person would be well advised to be more careful about indiscriminately downing thick steaks, potatoes drowned in butter, milk shakes and fried foods."

The same fatty foods that cause cancer will also cause arthritis. Senator George McGovern stated that at least seven out of ten major diseases are caused by faulty nutrition.

We are truly sorry to deprive you of the foods you have used and enjoyed for some time. However, we must be fair with you. Having found, after much study and testing, that certain foods are harmful to the human body, it is our duty to accurately report these findings to our readers, and this we have done.

To compensate for this, we have spent many hours formulating a collection of recipes and developing ingredients, which should take the place of those you are giving up. These special recipes and substitutes will satisfy the pleasure you take in eating, without being harmful to your health.

CHAPTER IV

NATURAL NUTRITION MOST ESSENTIAL IN THE PREVENTION AND TREATMENT OF ARTHRITIS

In spite of the fact that our health authorities and health agencies are telling the public that nutrition has no bearing on arthritis, I claim the opposite. I maintain that NUTRITION IS THE KEY TO THE SOLUTION OF THE ARTHRITIS PROBLEM. My conclusion is based on over half a century of study, research and personal experience. As a result, there is absolutely no doubt in my mind that: Nutrition is the most important approach to the solution of this problem.

The human body is composed of a number of organic chemical substances. These are continually being used up in the normal process of living (metabolism). To maintain normal good health, these components must be replenished through the foods we eat daily. That is why it is said, "We are what we eat." I would add also — "what we drink, what we breathe, and what we think."

It is exceedingly fortunate that the human body has the remarkable power of healing itself, even after years of abuse. This it can do only if it is given a healthful environment and fed *natural foods.*

There are two classes of foods — natural foods and denatured or processed foods. The natural foods are the only foods that will encourage life, promote strength and endurance, and help to restore lost health. Denatured or processed foods will always interfere with the normal functions of the body and, sooner or later, cause sickness and disease. You will find the natural foods close to nature — in the gardens, orchards and groves, tapping all the vital substances from the rain, soil, atmosphere and sunshine — combining these life-giving elements so that they will be exactly right for your digestive system. On the other hand, foods from factories are artificial.

There are thirty-seven million persons suffering with arthritis in the United States and the number is increasing each year. The reason for this is that people are using more and more processed foods. Statistics show that 65% of the food in our nation comes from factories. The food comes in cans, bottles, packages, etc. Also, a large percentage of meals are eaten in restaurnats, where the public has no control over the ingredients used.

THE BODY — A SENSITIVE INSTRUMENT

Most persons do not realize that the body is a very delicate instrument and a complex chemical laboratory. When we put any substance into it that was not designed by Nature as food for mankind, the entire process of metabolism is upset.

The average motorist is very careful about the type of fuel he puts into his automobile. He would not dream of trying to run his auto on water, or water mixed with gasoline, or pour into his car any other substance not intended as fuel.

But with his own precious body, which is, after all, a highly developed, complex and sensitive machine, the average person gives very little thought to the "fuel" he pours into it (as long as it tastes good) — no matter how unsuitable it may be. He buys and eats what the commercial food interests prepare and induce him to eat, through the art of advertising.

Eating these "foodless foods", so suitably called "junk foods", the average person knows not the injury he is doing to his precious body-machine, until, sooner or later, serious consequences result — disease, and finally, an early and painful death.

THE BASIC DIET CONTINUED

In Chapter II, the use of fruits in The Basic Diet was covered. In Chapter III, the substances you should eliminate from your diet were listed. We now continue to discuss the other components of *The Basic Diet*.

Fresh fruits, fresh vegetable salads, fresh nuts, seeds, whole grains, legumes and sprouts, should be the main ingredients of *The Basic Diet*. Meat is not included.

SALADS

Salads should make up an important part of your diet each day. Of all the various forms of lettuce, head lettuce is the easiest to digest. You can chop it fine on a breadboard. Butter lettuce is also easy to digest; romaine is harder to digest. However, romaine contains more chlorophyll.

USE OF RAW SPINACH

As a variation, it is good to use one part fresh, raw, chopped spinach to two parts lettuce, chopped. It's attractive, delicious, and healthful. (See the recipe section.)

USE OF RAW CABBAGE

A substitute for lettuce is raw cabbage, grated.

THE VALUE OF SALADS

Fresh vegetable salads are very important for vitamin and mineral content, nutritional value, and a laxative effect. The salad should be a really large one and form the main part of at least one meal every day. It should not be too complicated — two, three, or four ingredients are enough. A *large* salad, with half a ripe avocado (if available) and a baked or toasted potato (as described elsewhere), will make an ideal meal. A salad and one or two steamed vegetables is another simple, wholesome meal. Of course, you can always sprout seeds in your own kitchen, for salad greens.

LIQUID SALADS

Here is a salad variation you may not have thought of: put several raw vegetables, cut up, into your blender, and blend them well. Pour into a glass and drink, or eat with a spoon. This is a LIQUID SALAD, and it's full of vitamins, minerals and enzymes, because the vegetables are raw. It is an ideal food for babies and for the elderly with poor teeth and dentures, who cannot chew many raw vegetables. Actually, it is good for everyone. You can get many more raw vegetables "inside of you" this way, than when you have to chew them.

SALAD DRESSINGS

Salad dressings are very important. Therefore, it is essential to do a bit of research on their preparation and use. Choose one that appeals to your individual taste. The main thing to remember is to use healthful ingredients and to avoid the ordinary dressings in the supermarkets, most of which contain salt, sugar, preservatives and other additives. These are some of the offenders that are causing arthritis in increasing numbers. If you make your salad dressings at home, you'll know what they contain. See the sample dressings we have created and put into the recipe section.

SALAD VEGETABLES

Carrots	Celery	Cucumbers	Lettuce
Onions	Parsley	Radishes	Spinach
Sprouts	Tomatoes	Watercress	

Some of these should be eaten *liberally every day*. USE THEM RAW.

IMPORTANCE OF WARMING FOODS

It is very important not to eat your salads or other foods cold. The cold inhibits the actions of the enzymes, especially in the winter time. Warm your food a little before eating.

An example of the importance of eating warm, rather than cold, food, comes to mind:

Mrs. S. came to me complaining that she was lacking in energy and losing weight, for no apparent reason. After questioning her extensively about how she prepared her food, I learned that she was in the habit of taking foods from the refrigerator (salads, milk, juices, fruits, etc.), and immediately serving them, without warming them. I suggested that she stop this, and begin warming her foods before eating them. (Some foods naturally must be warmed in a saucepan; others, such as whole fruits, can be left in cupboards, and need not be in the refrigerator in the first place.)

She followed my advice, and the changes that took place in her health were surprising. Soon afterwards, she regained her energy and normal weight.

VEGETABLES

Most fresh vegetables are good, but CANNED VEGETABLES SHOULD BE STRICTLY AVOIDED, because they contain salt, white sugar, and chemical preservatives that are bad for anyone troubled with arthritis. They are dead foods.

Dr. Michael L. Gerber, M.D., a noted nutritional scientist, states that 93 percent of the vitamins, minerals and enzymes are destroyed in the canning process of foods.

The quality of fresh vegetables varies greatly, and one should learn to pick the best available. With a little study and extra attention, one can learn to judge quality. The ideal vegetable is organic (unsprayed) and picked shortly before eating. The logical conclusion to this fact is: have your own vegetable garden if you possibly can.

During the winter months, if fresh vegetables are not available, dried and frozen ones may be used, but *make sure they have not been seasoned with salt or sugar.* Form the habit of reading the labels to see if they have been treated with chemicals, preservatives, etc.

Everyone knows about the valuable Vitamin C in citrus fruits, but there is a vegetable that is a better source. It is bell peppers. A raw red pepper contains 190 mg. of vitamin C; a yellow pepper has 184 mg.; a green pepper has 89.3. The same amount of orange has a mere 53 mg. of vitamin C. The raw, red pepper is a beautiful and healthful addition to your daily salad; you can chop it fine, or cut it into strips. Yes, they are expensive, but watch for sales at your supermarket.

SPECIES OF VEGETABLES

Artichokes	Jerusalem Artichoke
Asparagus	Kale
Beets (with tops)	Kohlrabi
Bell Peppers (red are best)	Leeks
Broccoli	Lima Beans (fresh)
Brussels Sprouts	Mustard Greens
Cabbage	Okra
Cauliflower	Parsley
Celery	Peas
Chard	Potatoes
Chayote	Rutabaga
Chinese Cabbage	Scallions
Chives	Spinach
Collards	Squashes
Corn on the Cob	String Beans
Cucumbers	Sweet Peppers
Dandelion	Sweet Potatoes
Eggplant	Turnips (with tops)
Escarole	Watercress
Garlic	Yams

THE BEST WAYS TO PREPARE VEGETABLES

RAW:

Bell Pepper (grated)	Parsley
Carrots (whole; grated; blended)	Peas
Cauliflower (flowers only)	Radishes
Celery	Spinach
Cucumbers	Sprouts

BAKED:

Carrots	Squashes
Eggplant	Sweet Potatoes
Onions	Turnips
Potatoes	Yams

STEAMED:*

Asparagus	Peas
Broccoli**	Spinach
Carrots	Squashes
Cauliflower**	Swiss Chard**
Eggplant	Mushrooms

(* For information about steamers, see Chapter VI.)
(** Steam stems first)

BOILED:

Artichokes	Onions
Beets (with tops)	Parsley ***
Celery	Peas
Leeks	Potatoes
Lentils	String Beans
Lima Beans	Turnips

(***with other vegetables)

BROILED:

Bell Peppers	Sweet Potatoes
Mushrooms	Turnips
Potatoes	Yams

WITH VEGETABLES, THE LESS COOKING, THE BETTER

We mean not only in length of time, but in methods of preparation. Frying is the least desirable of all methods of preparing vegetables.

Cleanse your vegetables by immersing them in concentrated vinegar before eating or cooking, to rinse off any spray residues. Seek out organic produce.

SECONDARY FOODS

The above are the BASIC FOODS which I found to be agreeable in treating arthritis successfully, in my wife and others. These should be the *only foods used until all pain has gone.*

Other foods follow that you will wish to eat. But add these foods very cautiously, and *only one at a time.* Use them regularly for *two or three weeks,* and if they do not cause trouble, you may then feel free to eat them. If any of the symptoms of arthritis return, then they should be avoided.

CEREALS

Practically all the *packaged* cereals are flavored with salt, sugar, and malt, and these are very troublesome in cases of arthritis. The following five whole grain cereals are the ones we have found most satisfactory:

Buckwheat Groats (fine grind), *Millet, Rolled Oats* (if not chemically treated), *Whole Wheat* and *Brown Rice.*

BUCKWHEAT GROATS come in two forms: toasted and raw. The raw is rather hard to get, but is available in whole kernels. If you can get it, put it through a grinder; then either use it alone or combined half-and-half with the fine grind buckwheat groats, sometimes called "kasha."

Buckwheat is a favorite because, first, it contains rutin and other nutrients not found in the ordinary cereals. Secondly, it is the least starchy of all the grains, therefore less fattening and less mucus forming. Thirdly, it is a soft cereal and can be prepared without cooking it "to death."

Here is *the best way to prepare buckwheat groats:*

Use one part of the groats to 3 1/2 parts of water. (It's best to use only bottled water for drinking and cooking.) Use a Pyrex glass pot with a well-fitting cover. Boil the water briskly and slowly add the groats; then cover the pot and turn off the heat. Let the mixture stand for about five minutes. All the water will be absorbed by the cereal, and it will be soft and fluffy. Add a little honey and low-fat milk or soy milk and you will have a delicious, healthful dish.

HULLED MILLET is a protein cereal, and an excellent hot cereal for young and old, but being a *hard grain*, it requires more cooking than the buckwheat, which is a soft grain.

To prepare millet:

Use 3 1/2 parts water to one part millet. Cook slowly until the millet is soft and fluffy. Add honey or maple syrup and low-fat milk or soy milk.

ROLLED OATS make an easily digested cereal, which can be prepared with a minimum of cooking, the same as buckwheat. The only precaution is to look at the label and make sure the contents have not been treated with any chemical preservative.

WHOLE WHEAT: Buy the wheat "berries" in a health food store. Grind them in an electric grinder. It is a hard grain, and must be cooked well. Eat with honey and a little low-fat milk or soy milk.

BROWN RICE is much superior to white rice. It is the grain highest in B-complex vitamins, essential for healthy neurological function. Rice is quite high in starch, so it should not be used to excess. For a lunch or dinner, it can be combined with onions and green peppers, with which it combines nicely, and makes the mixture less concentrated in starch.

PREPARED CEREALS: You will find wholesome "cold" cereals in your health food store, some in bulk and some in packages. In the latter case, read the ingredients. Granola is a very tasty prepared cereal. Add soy milk from your health food store.

SOY SAUCE and TAMARI

Orientals eat much more rice than other people. They use soy sauce and tamari sauce, which are highly concentrated, salty seasonings, and a *great cause of arthritis.*

So, if rice is used, omit the soy and tamari sauce. Use avocado, onion, garlic, or one of the powdered seasonings described in this book.

NATURAL SOURCES OF PROTEIN

NUTS: Fresh raw nuts and seeds make excellent sources of protein. Most of the raw, fresh nuts may be used, but for those with arthritis, the almonds and sunflower seeds are best. However, they should never be eaten roasted and/or salted. Almonds should be blanched to remove the tough, brown skin.

An easy way to blanch almonds:

Drop the almonds into hot water, and let them stand for a few minutes in the covered pot. (If the skin comes off easily when the almond is squeezed, it is ready.) Pour off the hot water and remove the skins.

Store the blanched almonds in a sealed glass jar or a plastic bag in the refrigerator. You may wish to eat the almonds with fresh fruit (never use canned).

We purchase our nuts in the shell, year 'round, via mail order companies. This way, we can get organic nuts, fresh, that keep for a long time., and at an economical price. In fact, at this writing, we have a 50-pound bag of filberts in the shell in our pantry.

Beware all shelled nuts in stores. They have been subjected to all kinds of chemicals and dyes. Avoid buying blanched almonds. Nature provided the brown skin for protection, and when almonds are skinned, the "naked" nut can become rancid. You can easily blanch your almonds at home, as you need them. We leave the brown skins on, when grinding the almonds.

SEEDS: SUNFLOWER, SESAME

SUNFLOWER SEEDS are extremely rich in vitamins, minerals, and first class natural nutrients, but they must be fresh. The way to tell if they are fresh is to taste them. They should taste sweet in flavor. If they do not taste good, they are old and should not be used. Before using a quantity, we put some on a flat plate, look at them through a magnifying glass, and discard any defective ones.

Remember — *do not buy salted sunflower seeds.*

SESAME SEEDS are very rich in essential nutrients. In fact, they are nutritional powerhouses. They contain over 35% protein and have twice as much calcium as milk, and as much iron as liver. Purchase them unhulled from your health food store. They make a delicious confection when combined with almonds and honey. (See recipe for Carob Candy.) A good way to use the seeds is to put them through a grinder and sprinkle them over fresh fruit.

OILS: In cases of arthritis, *all other* oils besides olive oil should be avoided. We have tried others, and found them troublesome in cases of arthritis.

In buying olive oil, one should be very choosy, because much of the olive oil in the ordinary market has been kept in a warm environment and is thereby spoiled. It is important to get it as fresh as possible from the source and keep it in the refrigerator. In fact, all oils need to be stored in a refrigerator.

Virgin olive oil is the only oil that is truly "cold pressed." All vegetable oils are subjected to heat during the extraction process. In some cases, a chemical solvent is used to extract the oil, later driven off with heat.

Italians in their native land use olive oil instead of butter. It is cholesterol-free, and far more healthful.

LEGUMES: Lentils and lima beans are excellent protein foods. Dried beans should be soaked in hot water for several hours before cooking; lentils don't need soaking. Lentils combine well with onions, carrots, and celery.

The lima beans should be skinned before cooking. After soaking a few hours, the skins come off very easily. Combine with onions and tomatoes; for seasoning use garlic and a few bay leaves. (Use the extra large limas.)

A tip for bean recipes: add strips of Kombu, a common sea vegetable, to the pot. Kombu helps the beans to cook faster and to be digested more easily.

SPROUTS are an excellent form of protein. In addition, they are a very rich source of vitamins and minerals. (See Chapter V on "Sprouting Living Foods.")

Note: All of the above are concentrated forms of protein, but there is a certain amount of protein in all foods.

CARBOHYDRATES

BREAD: Most of the breads in the market are salted, and contain preservatives to keep them soft and "everlastingly" fresh. The salt and preservatives play havoc with arthritis. It is therefore advisable to be cautious. If possible, bake your own bread with whole grain flour and wholesome ingredients. If you cannot bake it yourself, visit your health food store and try to find a bread made of whole grain flour, soya flour or millet, honey and yeast. Read the ingredients to make sure the bread contains no salt, no white sugar, no white flour and no preservatives. Any *one* of these ingredients can perpetuate an arthritic condition indefinitely.

Thoroughly toasted bread is much better than fresh bread. A good way to prepare such toast is to cut each slice into four parts, then toast them *under the broiler until dark brown.* Turn the pieces over and toast the other sides the same way. Toasting the bread in *the ordinary toaster will not do*; it should be done under the broiler where the toasting penetrates through and through. This reduces the starch and lessens the effect of the salt, if there is salt in the bread. You can put these toasted pieces in a plastic bag and keep them in the cupboard for future use.

What about sandwiches? Made with fresh bread, they are an item you should delete from your diet. Fresh bread is very mucus-forming.

Anyone who wants to get rid of arthritis, or prevent it, should not eat bread with jam or with ordinary salted butter. The better way is to eat the toasted bread with avocado — with or without a little honey.

POTATOES: Here is one of the best foods for combating arthritis. Eaten without butter, potatoes are not fattening. They are versatile in that they may be baked, boiled in a stew, or toasted. From a nutritional standpoint, it is better to eat toasted potatoes instead of bread.

TOASTED POTATOES:

Use the large size Idaho, Russet or White Rose potatoes. First peel the potatoes, then cut into slices about 1/4 inch thick. Spread the slices on a large metal pan. Place the pan under the broiler, then broil the slices until they begin to blister. Turn the slices over and toast the other sides until these begin to blister. This takes very little time.

A little sweet butter, soy margarine or avocado may be spread over the slices. The potato prepared this way is tasty and nutritious — much more so than bread. For an *excellent menu idea,* this toasted potato — served with a large salad — makes an ideal meal for anyone. *Simplicity* is an important principle in food preparation. The simpler the meal, the easier it is to digest.

BAKED POTATOES

Here is an ideal way to bake potatoes:

First, you must have a heavy cast iron pot with a well fitting cover. Depending on the size of the pot, it will accommodate from one to four potatoes. To bake the potatoes *on top of the stove quickly,* simply place your unpeeled potatoes in the pot, without any water. (If potatoes are large, you may cut them in half.) Turn the heat up high to start with. Turn down to medium when well heated. It should then take very little time to complete the baking — from five to ten minutes.

This is a quick method, and as you do not use the oven, you do not heat the whole kitchen because of a few potatoes baking for an hour. *Yams, sweet potatoes, and onions* can also be baked this way.

Toasted or baked potatoes are excellent for settling an upset stomach.

DAIRY PRODUCTS

Dairy products are not part of the *Basic Diet*, but they may be added one at a time after the pain of arthritis is gone.

Here are some *Cardinal Rules* regarding dairy products:

MILK: Instead of whole milk, it is best to use low-fat or skim milk, which is less fattening, less mucus-forming, and less cholesterol-forming.

Persons who are vegans (using no animal by-products) now use one of the new, non-dairy milks made of soy beans or rice, available in health food stores.

BUTTER: Butter should be sweet, *unsalted*. Most of the butter sold is salted. It keeps better with less spoilage, so the food vendors favor it. But salted butter is "murder" for all cases of arthritis. So make sure the butter you use is *unsalted*. As with *whole* milk, butter is fattening and a potent cause of cholesterol, so it should be used *sparingly*. Also, note that sweet butter is more perishable, so keep it in the *freezer* compartment of your refrigerator.

For *weight control,* use more *avocados* and less butter. Avocados can be used in many places instead of butter. *One pound* of avocado will add less weight than *one ounce* of butter. So do not be afraid to use the avocado, which is truly a health food.

Health food stores now offer margarine made of soy beans, a good substitute for butter.

CHEESE: Almost all the cheeses in the market are highly salted and are often treated with preservatives and additives—causes of arthritis.

Soy cheese is now available in health food stores, a good alternative.

Would you believe that Plaster of Paris is added to cottage cheese to make it stiff? When I first heard about this outlandish practice, I did not believe it, so I telephoned one of my patients who worked in a dairy. He confirmed the fact: "Plaster of Paris is being used in commercial cottage cheese." I then set out to find a substitute for the commercial cheeses, and developed a home-made cottage cheese that is easy to make and delicious to taste.

Practically all the commercial cheeses contain salt, artificial coloring and additives — inducing arthritis.

Homemade Cottage Cheese

Use a large glass or earthenware bowl. To two quarts of buttermilk, add the juice of one large lemon. Place the mixture in the oven under *very low heat*, the lowest possible. In four or five hours the buttermilk will form a thick clabber and separate from the whey. Pour the entire mixture into a cheesecloth bag, hang the bag over a bowl, and allow the whey to drain into the bowl. The remainder in the cheesecloth bag is a fine, delicious, delicate cheese, better than any you can buy. Place in a glass jar and store in the refrigerator. Do not discard the whey. It can be used as a nourishing drink, in soups or in salads.

A good recipe for using this homemade cottage cheese follows:

CREAMY DILL DRESSING

1 cup home-made cottage cheese
1/4 cup low-fat milk or soy milk
2 teaspoons dill weed powder
1 teaspoon lemon juice or cider vinegar
2 tablespoons olive oil
1/2 teaspoon kelp or dulse
1/2 teaspoon onion powder
1/2 teaspoon garlic powder

Put all ingredients into blender container. Cover and blend on high until smooth.

EGGS: Eggs should be *fresh*. They should not be seasoned with salt. Instead, they can be scrambled with chopped, sautéed onions. If you wish a soft-boiled or poached egg, you may sprinkle on it any of the salt substitutes mentioned in Chapter III.

In the vegetarian* literature widely available today, the true facts about egg production are revealed, and eggs are shown to be an unwholesome food. Truly, they are not necessary in a healthful diet. Americans are consuming too much protein.

If you buy eggs at a health food store, you will get a better quality egg, from free-roaming chickens who have not been fed drugs, and have had wholesome feed. Commercial eggs in the markets are from battery chickens who are given drugs in their feed, who are crowded, and otherwise treated inhumanely. Many are diseased.

PRECAUTIONS IN USING FRUITS AND VEGETABLES

If you want first-class health, you must choose first-class foods.

THE RIPENESS OF FRUIT

Fruits should be sweet, ripe, of good quality, and taste good. So many of the fruits in the markets are picked while still hard. These unripe fruits are poor in nutritional value and lacking in good flavor. Color, taste and smell are the best indicators of quality; the more color, the better the taste and food value, provided the fruits are organic. However, there are other elements to be considered besides color. Supermarket fruits often look beautiful but they are embalmed.

---

*Persons who do not consume flesh foods (meat, fish) are called *vegetarians*. Those who also eliminate animal by-products (eggs, milk, cheese) are called *vegans*.

There are certain times of the year when each fruit is in season and matures to its proper nutritional value. It is important to learn to judge foods, especially fruits. If the fruit is tasteless, too hard or sour, it should not be eaten. When shopping, buy one piece of fruit and taste it. If it tastes sweet and ripe, buy more.

However, if only unripe fruit is available, you have no choice. Do not put such fruit into your refrigerator — it will never ripen! This is very important. *Instead, put the fruit into a cupboard at room temperature,* and give it enough time to soften and ripen before eating.

SPRAYED FRUIT

Good fruit is fragrant. If the fruit smells of chemicals, you can be sure it has been heavily sprayed with insecticides. Since so many of the fruits are sprayed and waxed, it is best to peel all fruits not organically grown, before eating. These chemicals are very powerful and penetrating; they cannot be merely washed off as some persons think.

Also, whenever possible, you should find a source where you can buy *organically-grown fruits and vegetables.* Try to find a farm or even a small orchard where you can get your product at the source. Most health food stores have a produce section.

In some cities, there are CO-OPS; you become a member and shareholder. Here you can get organic produce. If there is none in your city, you might help to form one.

This is *very important,* so we are repeating it here. TRY TO OBTAIN FRUITS THAT ARE ORGANICALLY GROWN, WITHOUT PESTICIDES. THESE CHEMICALS CAN CAUSE A GREAT DEAL OF TROUBLE — arthritis and other illnesses — SO DO ALL YOU CAN TO LOCATE A SOURCE OF ORGANIC FRUIT. There are a few mail order sources.

ORANGES

Note that *all* unripe citrus fruits harm the tooth enamel and the intestinal tract lining, so watch the oranges you buy and eat.

It is customary now for the big citrus growers to treat (embalm) their fruits with a biphenol compound. My first experience with this problem occurred a number of years ago before I ever knew about this process of treating fruits.

My wife and I had eaten some oranges from the supermarket. Shortly afterwards, we both began to itch, mostly on the chest and nose. It did not take me long to conclude that the oranges had been treated, because this was the only food we both had eaten. I returned to the supermarket and asked the produce man to show me the box in which these oranges were packed. Upon close examination, I finally found a sentence, in very small print, which stated: "This fruit has been treated with biphenol to preserve its freshness." I asked the produce man about this. He had never heard of the process nor knew anything about it. Then I talked with the girl at the fresh juice bar in the supermarket. She was squeezing these same oranges. I asked her whether she knew anything about this chemical. She told me she did not. However, she added that she had to wear rubber gloves to protect her hands when cutting and handling the oranges. If she did not wear the gloves her hands would swell and itch. I then informed her about the printing on the box.

Biphenol is a chemical which is used to embalm living matter and is extremely bad for the human body.

Do not use orange peel or lemon peel in your recipes, unless the fruit is organically grown.

PREPARE YOURSELF FOR A SHOCK!

While we were writing this section for a new edition, we got the idea of tracking down more information on the chemical biphenol. If they use it to embalm our fruits, could it possibly be the same chemical that is used to embalm corpses in preparation for a good appearance in the casket at the funeral?

I telephoned a local mortuary, which confirmed that this was so. I was given the number of the chemical company, which further confirmed it: "YES, IT IS BIPHENOL THAT IS USED EXTENSIVELY IN THE EMBALMING PROCESS IN MORTUARIES"!

It is unbelievable what they are doing to the food today. You should do *everything* you *can* to *protect* yourself! Also do whatever you can to stop such practices, and join organizations that are working against food adulteration.

Is it any wonder that millions of Americans have cancer and arthritis?

SUPERMARKET FRUITS VS. ORGANIC FRUITS

Besides the embalming of fruit, dyes are also used to enhance the appearance of supermarket fruits. The biphenol, the dyes and all chemicals are harmful to the human body, especially in cases of arthritis.

You can now understand why the beautiful-looking fruits in our supermarkets are not what they appear to be. A red but hard peach, for example, is a deception. Not the sunshine, but gassing, produced the color. Peel such fruit. It is a good idea to be more suspicious of perfect-looking fruit than of the ordinary-looking fruit. Organically-grown fruits, as a rule, are not perfect in appearance because the natural elements, like sunshine, have made them rustic-looking. Even an occasional worm in an apple is an advantage instead of otherwise. In my younger days, I was horrified when I encountered a worm in my fruit. But now that I seldom see one, and know why, I welcome the occasional worm I encounter, for if the worm survives, I know I will. I know it is an organic fruit.

GROWING YOUR OWN

If you can have your own vegetable garden and a few fruit trees (this is possible even in a backyard), you have a real advantage.

You can leave the fruit on the tree until it is fully ripened. If the birds present a problem and try to take the fruit before you do, then drape cheesecloth over the tree, closing the lower ends with clothespins.

If you live in a cold climate and thus have months without access to much fresh produce, but have your own garden, you can get a home dryer and dry your excess fruits. Drying preserves more of the food values than freezing. The water in the fruit is evaporated and what you have left is a concentrated fruit form. Later, when you need to use it, you add water and reconstitute the fruit.

NO SYNTHETIC FRUIT PRODUCTS: There is a product on the market which claims to be "as good as real orange juice." It is *nothing but chemicals*; do not use it! Learn to read the labels.

NO SUGAR WITH FRUIT: *When sweetening fruit that is tart, such as grapefruit, use honey as a sweetener, not sugar, white or brown.*

MILK WITH FRUITS: It is important to make your food taste good. Quite a number of the fruits combine well with honey and low-fat milk. Low-fat milk is less fattening and less cholesterol-forming than whole milk. However, we now have other choices in the health food stores — non-dairy milks made of soy beans or rice, flavored with vanilla or carob.

YOUR TASTE BUDS ARE YOUR TEST BUDS

Recently, I prepared some organic Swiss chard a friend had given us. As instructed in this book, I cut off and steamed the stems first, as they take a bit longer to become soft, and then added the leaves. However, the leaves were too bitter for me, and I did not eat them. I do not believe in eating anything that does not taste good, even if it is supposed to be good for you.

YOUR TASTE BUDS ARE YOUR "TEST BUDS"! Nature has given them to you to screen out foods that are not good for you. Mankind has largely lost this instinct. For example, tobacco and alcohol at first taste bitter and unpleasant. But if a person persists in using them, they get hold of him, and addictions set in. Bitter and bad-tasting though they may be, people like the effects they give. The people are addicted, "hooked," victims of a bad, unhealthful habit. If they had paid attention to their taste buds the first time, realizing that Nature was trying to protect them from harm, this would not have happened.

OTHER FRUITS

PEARS: There are many varieties of pears on the market that are poor in quality. Color and taste will help you determine which is the best. The Winter Nellis is a favorite, then the Comica and Bartlett.

LEMONS: Lemons, of course, are sour but, even so, they should be *ripe* and used mainly in salads in combination with olive oil. Too much lemon juice hurts tooth enamel and also damages the lining of the intestinal tract. So always use olive oil with lemon juice. In warm weather, if lemonade is desired, prepare it with honey, not sugar.

PINEAPPLES: Sometimes you see in the supermarkets unripe fresh pineapples. They are green on the outside. These you may buy, as they will ripen in a warm place in your home. However, sometimes the supermarket will cut them in half, and then *they will never ripen!* So, do not buy green, unripe, cut pineapples!

BERRIES: A large percentage of berries are sour, as they are picked unripe. Only the vine-ripened berries are sweeter, and even then most berries have a natural sour taste.

If you wish to eat berries, add a little low-fat milk or soy or rice milk and honey, but never sugar.

Fruits like cranberries and rhubarb need a great amount of sweetening to make them edible. It is not advisable to use much of these fruits.

BANANAS: This is an excellent fruit, usually low in price and generally available. You may purchase bananas green in the markets, but allow enough time at home to ripen—wait until they are speckled. A warm place will hasten the ripening. They are excellent for all ages; a mashed, ripe banana is an ideal food for babies.

Although bananas are gassed at the source (to hasten ripening) we do not consider this harmful, as they have a thick skin and are always peeled.

FIGS: In addition to fresh fruits, you can use dates and dried fruits for naturally sweet desserts.

We use Black Mission figs (natural, organic, not sulphured or sprayed). Figs are 40% higher in dietary fiber than oatmeal, and almost three times as high as raisins, reports the California Fig Institute. They are also 80% higher in potassium than bananas, and *higher in calcium than whole milk!*

What's more, they are very low in sodium, virtually fat free (only one gram of fat per 100 grams of figs), and contain no cholesterol at all.

DATES: Dates may be called "the candy that grows on trees." The date is quite possibly the world's perfect, natural dessert. It is mankind's oldest domesticated fruit, and is used as a staple food in countries like Morocco, where dates originated. In fact, millions of people use them as the principal item of diet. Those people who travel by camel find them ideal; light to carry, and non-perishable in the desert.

Unsurpassed as a quick source of energy, they have many vitamins and minerals. The calorie count is very low—only 24 calories for an average-size date. Dates are:

High in fiber	No sodium
Rich in iron	No cholesterol
High in potassium and magnesium	No Fat

If you have children, we urge you to give them these wholesome, natural sweets, instead of candy made of sugar, chocolate, and other harmful substances. Young children can be easily taught to enjoy the natural foods. Also, use dates in your baking recipes, instead of sugar.

RAISINS: Made from grapes. California grapes are heavily sprayed, and there may be more chemicals used in preparation of raisins. Seek out organic raisins, sun-dried.

SPECIAL NOTE

WE URGE YOU TO PEEL ALL FRUITS AND VEGETABLES THAT CAN BE PEELED, TO AVOID MOST OF THE PESTICIDE RESIDUES — UNLESS YOU ARE SURE THEY ARE ORGANIC AND FREE FROM PESTICIDES.

NATURE'S CONFECTIONS

Honey	Dates	Raisins, Figs, Sun-dried	Prunes
Apricots	Peaches	Apples	Pears, etc.

Use Nature's confections instead of the artificial, sugary concoctions from the factories and bakeries.

Dried figs, prunes and raisins are very often treated with chemicals. It is therefore important to use these with caution. If after eating any of these your pain returns, you should stop using them. That is why this plan recommends adding these supplementary foods *one at a time*. In that way you can find out which foods are good for you and which are not. Again, seek out organic food sources.

NUTS AND SEEDS, SUGGESTIONS

Nuts and seeds are an important source of protein. Both are perishable foods, and if they are kept in a warm place for any length of time they will spoil. Most people, including the storekeepers, are not aware of this fact, and as a result a high percentage of the nuts and seeds in the stores are spoiled and not good to eat. This is especially true during the latter part of the year when the supply of nuts has been kept through the warm summer months.

When you go to buy these foods it is well to observe certain precautions. During the months of August, September, October and November, the old crop of nuts is still in the stores and for that reason you should be cautious not to buy any which may be spoiled because of improper storage. The best way to tell if they are good or not is to taste them. They should be pleasant to the taste. If they do not taste good they should not be eaten. By observing this precaution, and with a little experience, you will soon learn to pick nuts and seeds that are satisfactory for consumption.

Another suggestion to observe: Avoid salted and roasted nuts and seeds. Use only the fresh raw nuts. There are a number of nuts that may be used but our favorite is the almond, and our favorite seed the sunflower seed. People with poor teeth should grind these foods in an electric grinder and combine them with fresh fruits. It is best to purchase nuts in the shell, for freshness. Nature has provided a "coat of armor" with the shells. Take advantage of this protection.

If you purchase a large sack at one time (in large cities, nut dealers sell 50-lb bags), buy the new crop, not a bag from the old crop.

MEATS

You will note that the flesh foods — meat, poultry and fish — have not been listed in the Basic Diet for arthritis. Some arthritis sufferers report that these foods have adverse effects.

The chemicals used in the feeding and processing of the animals and chickens most likely cause the troubles.

These chemicals interfere with the normal functions of the body and cause much pain. If you must have flesh foods, try to get so-called organic meat which has not been treated with chemicals. They are available in some health food stores.

If you wish to include these flesh foods in your diet, then I suggest that you first adhere to the Basic Diet until your pain subsides. Then slowly add these flesh foods to your diet, and watch carefully to see how they affect your condition. If they cause the pain to return, you will have to act accordingly.

FISH

If you want to include fish in your diet, try adding it after the pain subsides. Do not add salt or white flour while preparing.

All canned fish is heavily salted and treated with preservatives.

Remember that fish is a very perishable food; make sure it is fresh. Actually, it is difficult to find fish that is fresh enough, in stores.

If you are concerned about getting an adequate supply of protein, remember that the following foods will serve you well in your protein needs: nuts, seeds, beans, peas, lentils, and sprouts. Actually, Americans and other Western people over-eat on protein, tremendously.

BELIEVE IT OR NOT — NUTRITION IS THE KEY!

You have been told again and again, by your doctors and the health agencies, that "nutrition (diet) has nothing to do with arthritis."

My research on this subject, extending for over 50 years, has convinced me, on the contrary, that NUTRITION IS THE KEY TO THE SOLUTION OF THIS SERIOUS PROBLEM!

Now, I have given you a well-rounded selection of natural foods which I have tested and retested to make sure they are beneficial for those troubled with arthritis. The main cause of arthritis is an unnatural, toxic diet. There are other causes but, in the majority of cases, the diet is the important factor. It would be a good idea to consult with your doctor to see if there are any other causes that need correction.

I have devoted over 50 years *researching and living* this subject. I do not know of anybody else who has gone into this important health matter more thoroughly than I have. Not only have I had the advantage of observing thousands of cases of arthritis, but I have gone so far as to purposely produce arthritis in my own body, and then get rid of it by employing the procedures presented in this manual. In just two weeks I can actually produce the symptoms of arthritis in my own body by eating an *unnatural, toxic diet*, and in a week or two be rid of the pain and other symptoms of arthritis by eating *natural foods*.

During my fifty years as a practicing dentist, many arthritis patients came to me with advice from their physicians to have their teeth extracted (as I stated before). I saw that this practice was not warranted. I would X-ray their teeth, and if they looked good I would leave them alone and advise the patient to adopt the diet I have here outlined. The results were dramatic! In many cases the dreadful, piercing pain would subside in a week or two. It seems incredible that so terrible a disease as arthritis can be relieved so easily, and yet it is so hard for our medical people to recognize and adopt this method. One of the reasons for this may be the fact that our medical students receive very little, if any, nutritional training. Some years ago, the drug industry took the helm of the entire medical field, including the curricula of medical schools.

So, dear reader, I want you to realize and understand that what I am giving you here is *not* some theory that may or may not be sound — that may or may not work — but rather, a thoroughly tested and retested plan that works with gratifying results — IF ADHERED TO!

ARTHRITIS IN CHILDREN

Once arthritis was a disease of the elderly. Now children have it! What has caused this? Is there some mysterious, malicious virus which once attacked only the mature and elderly, but now has decided to attack the young also? By no means. That would be superstition. The "mystery" is solved and the answer is crystal clear.

Nowadays, babies are fed on canned baby foods, with their harmful ingredients of sugar, salt, and chemical additives. By the time they are six or so, in many cases these substances, which have no place in the human body, have affected the bones and joints. After baby foods, the children eat the other harmful foods (the American "junk-food" diet).

Once we watched a television show on arthritis appealing for funds for research. The entire program showed young children who were suffering from arthritis. It was truly heart-rending to see children, as young as six, unable to run and play. They were afflicted with crippling arthritis.

The methods of treatment were drugs, inoculations with "gold shots," casts, and the use of warm water. (We can only approve of the warm water.) Not a word was said about the diet these children are on! It is a tragic situation, with all that needless suffering of the helpless young.

One little girl was interviewed about her arthritis. She said, in her little baby voice, "The doctor gave me Valium, and the next day I couldn't walk!" This indicates that no cure is found in drugs, which can only aggravate the situation, sometimes critically.

Even if you do not have children, please do all you can to spread this information — that the principal cause of arthritis is the additives in today's foods (plus the common "three bad whites"), and the answer is to change the diet to a wholesome, natural one!

We have already written on the harmfulness of sugar, but will repeat it here in this section on "arthritis in children." Would you feed your child candy for breakfast? No, yet millions of American mothers are doing practically that when they serve their children the highly-advertising sugar-coated cereals. These foods are more like candy than cereal. Pre-sweetened cereals contain from 30 to 50 percent sugar! So, right away, the first thing in the morning, the child who eats this food, is getting huge doses of this ingredient, sugar, that harms both the teeth and the general health. It also causes the child to feel filled, when he has not had sufficient good, wholesome food — food that builds bodies. Sugary foods give one the illusion of being well-fed, but later such food consumption will cause various illnesses and diseases, such as arthritis.

A survey shows what persuasive advertising can do. A study by the Texas A & M University System discovered that children's requests add 1.5 billion dollars per year to the American mother's grocery bills. You can be sure that these children are not seeing on television, and begging their mothers to buy, fruits and vegetables!

OTHER FACTORS THAT WILL HELP YOU OBTAIN OPTIMUM BENEFITS

Nutrition is of prime importance in combating arthritis, but there are other factors which will help you to obtain optimum benefits. I will discuss the three most important ones here.

FRESH AIR: The first of these is Fresh Air. During these times when smog and air pollution is so widespread, it is important to do all you can to live where the air is fresh. You have four choices — the country, the desert, the mountains or the seashore.

In addition, you should consider the quality of the air right in your own home where you live and sleep. Many, many homes are filled with polluted air as a result of sewer gas and also unvented gas stoves and gas heaters. If possible, use electricity for heating.

If there is a smoker in your home, try to have as much ventilation as you can. It would be better if the smoker would smoke outdoors or, better still, give up the habit.

Fresh air is the first essential of health. Without it, one cannot have good health. So do give this some thought. There is much, much more to say on this subject. Fresh air is the "first essential" of health and discussed in detail in our work *The Seven Essentials of Health.**

EXERCISE is another essential that must be considered if you want quick results. Exercise helps the circulation of blood and limbers up the joints of the body. Both of these are important in cases of arthritis. A good long walk and five or ten minutes of simple exercises daily will help one get quicker results in combating arthritis.

SUNSHINE — properly used — is of *tremendous* importance in combating arthritis. Besides supplying the body with the important Vitamin D, it causes the body to perspire. Through perspiration, the body gets rid of toxic matter. This is of prime importance.

Grace got rid of arthritis in the summertime. She would go on the roof of our apartment house in New York City, sunbathe (covering her head), and perspire profusely. This hastened her recovery markedly. Remember, your two allies in combating arthritis are (1) nutrition and (2) elimination. Perspiration is one channel of elimination through the skin.

By now you can realize that by ridding the body of arthritis, you will give the entire body a new lease on life. This has been the experience of many of those who have adopted this natural way of eating and living.

---

*To be republished by Tree of Life Publications

RECAPITULATION

Let us summarize briefly the important steps in combating arthritis.

1. THE CLEANSING PROCESS

RID THE BODY OF THE TOXIC MATTER which caused arthritis, using:

(A) Enemas/Colonics/Colemics; (B) Laxative Foods

2. DIET CONTROL

A. Mono-Diet of one or two foods (such as seedless grapes; watermelon; fresh, ripe pineapple; apples, pears; bananas; fresh carrot juice). *Eat only one or two at a time.* The pain should subside, then —

B. *Gradually* include the *Natural Foods* in the *Basic Diet.*

If any pain recurs, it means that one or more of the foods you are eating contains some chemical your body is rejecting. Limit your diet in the beginning, and by adding *one food at a time* you can easily identify the one which brought back the pain. Eliminate that food and the pain should leave. This careful selection of individual foods is a very effective way of finding out what foods are good for your individual case. This is very important.

Pain is Nature telling you that something you are doing or eating is wrong, and by the simple plan above, you can detect the offending food.

In time, you will have a good selection of foods that agree with you, and you are then on the road to recovery.

3. OTHER ESSENTIALS

Now you should help your body rejuvenate itself by adopting the *other Essentials of Health*, such as: (A) *Fresh Air;* (B) *Exercise;* (C) *Sunshine;* (D) *Water* (the use of water in healing is called Hydrotherapy). These are discussed on previous pages, and more thoroughly in our other work, *The Seven Essentials of Health.*

In this treatise, I have given you the knowledge it has taken me over fifty years to learn. It would be well for you to read, and carefully re-read the contents. If you will do this, and adopt the suggestions herein, I feel confident that you will be well rewarded with a more comfortable body, a better life — a LIFE FREE FROM SUFFERING!

AN IMPORTANT REMINDER

All the above may seem complicated, but as you adopt the natural diet and give these important instructions attention, you will soon learn how to nourish yourself properly, automatically, without giving it another thought.

Those who live in areas where the food supply is limited and meager need not despair. With the use of sprouts and a very few staple vegetables that are available all year around, one can nourish the body and help overcome arthritis.

Also, it is easy to obtain many health foods from companies who sell by mail. (See p. 250.) If you are unable to obtain some of the foods we have listed — do not feel discouraged. *Where there is a will, there is a way.*

THE HEALING POWER OF FASTING

Without a doubt, the fastest way to get rid of arthritis is through fasting. However, most people find it difficult and are not prepared to do this. They are afraid, and don't know how.

Arthritis sufferers could advantageously fast for one to three days (no food, only pure water), and then go on a mono-diet (one food at a time), as suggested in the plan of this book.

All long fasts should be done under the supervision of a health practitioner who is trained along this line.

To order a list of fasting institutions, see page 249.

The main point is what you do after the fast. If you go back to the old eating habits, the arthritis will return. The answer is a natural diet with as much uncooked foods as possible — salads, vegetables, sprouts, fruits, nuts, and seeds. And the diet should be made up of pure, unprocessed foods.

HOW TO COPE WITH HIGH FOOD PRICES

During a talk show, the interviewer asked: "How does the average person cope with the high prices charged in health food stores?"

I replied: "Assuming that nothing can be done about the high prices, it is better to pay a few dollars more for good food than give it to the doctor!" However, there are several ways to lower your costs of natural, healthful foods.

(1) Several families can join together to buy their foods wholesale.

(2) Your community may have a Co-Op for produce and other foods and items. If not, it can be started. There is a Co-Op Association.

(3) In Santa Monica, California, there are Farmers' Market days, twice a week, conducted by the city. Other cities have these. If yours does not, try suggesting it to City Hall.

(4) Try to grow some of your own food. A small yard is sufficient, or you can find a small, local grower who has more than he needs.

(5) Resort to the wonderful practice of sprouting seeds, which remarkably increases their vitamin and mineral values. Wheat, for example, has much more food value sprouted than when baked in bread, etc. In addition to increasing the food value and having health foods always on hand, the cost of sprouts is very low.

(6) Buy as many foods as you can in bulk instead of packaged. Packaging costs money. Often the cost of the package is more than the cost of its contents.

(7) When you do buy foods other than in bulk, it is not necessary to buy *name brands*. You are paying for the expensive advertising.

(8) Use fruits and vegetables when in season. Then the supply is greater than the demand; as a result, prices drop drastically.

(9) Patronize a merchant who is efficient and knows how to buy at a lower cost, thereby selling his merchandise at a lower cost. If he sells the same item as another for less, he is efficient and knows how to buy.

(10) Check the prices in different stores. They may vary tremendously for the same item. One merchant may be marking up the price exorbitantly.

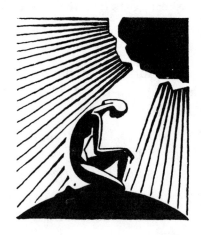

"Nature never did betray
The heart that loved her."

CHAPTER V

SPROUTING LIVING FOODS FOR A HEALTHIER LIFE

This chapter on sprouts is being added to this edition because of its great importance to all who are serious about regaining and retaining good health. It is of special importance to those who reside where a good supply of fresh fruits and fresh vegetables is not available, and to those who cannot afford to pay for fresh, organically-grown fruits and vegetables.

Marci Cohen, an authority on sprouting, who is teaching school children in Los Angeles how to sprout seeds, gives an interesting lecture on "How to Grow Your Living Food Indoors." She begins her talk with the following remarks:

"Do you know that a small corner in your house or apartment can produce more healthful, nutritious food than acres of chemically-sprayed crops? Sprouts and greens can be grown at home at any time of the year, in any weather, most economically, without soil and with very little water.

"Sprouts are a complete food with enzymes, minerals, trace elements, vitamins and complete proteins."

Dr. Ann Wigmore, a noted authority on sprouts and general health (retained or regained through *natural* ways) is the Founder and Director of the Ann Wigmore Foundation in Boston and Puerto Rico. Here some remarkable healing is being done of cancer and other serious ailments, by teaching the guests how to make living food the main part of their diet. It is not a hospital or clinic, but a school where health instruction is given.

In her excellent book *Garden Indoors — A New Concept in Diet,"* Dr. Wigmore gives us a fine summary on "Why and How to Sprout," which follows:

"Sprouting can be great fun and a real adventure. It can provide your family with nutritious food both summer and winter and cost pennies per meal. It is a wise, nutritional hobby that will pay for itself many times over. Sprouts are full of vitamins, minerals and quantities of easily digested protein, and can replace your fruits and vegetables because sprouts contain the elements these foods have and often much more. Sprouted seeds are an excellent source of Vitamins A, B-Complex, D, D, E, G, K, and even U, and minerals such as calcium, magnesium, phosphorus, chlorine, potassium, sodium and silicon, all in natural forms which the body can assimilate.

"Organic seeds can furnish so much Vitamin C that the eating of fruit for this purpose is unnecessary.

"Dr. Pauline Berry Mack of the University of Pennsylvania tested soybeans for Vitamin C content and discovered that, when sprouted for 72 hours, one-half cup of these shoots contained as much Vitamin C as six glasses of orange juice.

"Dr. Paul Burkholder of Yale University discovered that oats sprouted for five days contained 500% more B6, 600% more folic acid, 10% more B1 and 1350% more B2 than unsprouted oats.

"Dr. Loa of Yenching University in Peking reports that the high level of simple sugars in sprouts makes the little shoots an excellent 'quick energy' food. And your cost for this delicious, vitamin-packed food is less than 5 cents per pound.

"The first step in sprouting is to be sure the seed you purchase is organically grown and has not been sprayed or chemically treated in any way. Chemicals can damage the embryo and cause the seed to rot instead of sprout. And, of course, these chemicals will poison you, too. Almost any seed or grain or legume can be successfully sprouted, although most devotees prefer alfalfa, soybeans, mung beans and lentils, and the cereal grasses — wheat, oats, rye and barley. Unhulled sesame and sunflower seeds, radish, mustard, red clover, fenugreek, corn, lima beans, pinto and kidney beans, chick peas and nearly any other seed can be sprouted successfully. However, potato sprouts should never be eaten, as the plant is a member of the deadly nightshade family.

"Almost any kind of container can be used successfully for your sprout garden. We use half-gallon wide mouth jars such as you would use for canning, and one-gallon wide mouth jars for larger mixtures of seeds. Cut out or remove the inner surface of the lid and insert a piece of wire screening or cheesecloth in double thickness in its place. Or if you prefer, simply secure screening or cheese cloth with a rubber band. Another idea is an earthenware flower pot with its bottom drain hole covered by cheesecloth or wire screening or even a wad of cotton. Unglazed pottery is excellent as it absorbs water and thus insures that the shoots will be kept moist, but not wet. Cover pot with a saucer, but not too tightly as sprouts need ventilation, and set it in a shallow pan or saucer. Even an ordinary bowl works if you carefully drain the seeds after each rinsing. Experiment with your equipment according to your own resources and needs.

"Pick out any chaff, cracked seeds or hulls and check the seeds for fertility (sterile seeds will float). Wash your seeds thoroughly and put into jar or container. Use one cup of such seeds as lentils, mung beans, chick peas, and one to three tablespoons of the smaller, finer seeds, such as alfalfa or radish. Now fill the jar with water and let the seeds soak overnight. The soak water should be warm, of room temperature, and free from chlorine or fluorine, which can interfere with the sprouting process. Use spring or distilled water.

"Next morning, pour off the water and drink it or save it to add to juices or soup stock. It is loaded with water-soluble vitamins and minerals. Rinse seeds carefully and place them in your dish rack (with the jar top down at a 45 degree angle) for a short while to insure proper drainage of sprouts. Then place the jar in a warm environment, preferably on its side so the seeds will have better ventilation, and where you can see it so you won't forget to tend your sprouts. In the evening, rinse the seeds again to keep them moist and during the next few days be sure to keep the seeds moist by rinsing and draining them morning and night.

"In about three days, you will see the seeds produce tiny sprouts. They are ready to be eaten when they have sprouted fully. They are at their peak of vitamin potency 60 to 90 hours after germinating. Grain sprouts should be eaten when very short, about the length of the kernel, or they become bitter. Sunflower sprouts also develop a rather unpleasant taste when they exceed the length of the seed. Soybeans, peas and alfalfa are about right when their sprouts are from two to three inches long. Each has its own distinctive flavor; there is a great potential for variety to suit each personal taste. To prevent them from growing too much after sprouting, for they are tender when young, after exposing them to the light until they are chlorophyll-rich green, refrigerate them until they are all used. They will keep for several days.

"There is no limit to the ways in which sprouts can be tastily prepared to yield their nutritional treasure. Sprouts can be eaten by anyone with a health problem, for they are readily digested. There is as much variety in the taste of sprouts as there is in traditional vegetables. Personal tastes vary, starting with fresh, raw salads, which yield the optimum vitamin content of sprouts. Rye sprouts add a mouth-watering wild rice tang when sprinkled into soups just before serving. And they make an excellent snack and pick-me-up beverage."

Catharyn Elwood packs many examples into a few pages of her book *Feel Like a Million* (Pocket Books, New York). We quote from this book:

"With less really fertile farm land, and a minimum of modern farm machinery, China feeds nearly one billion of its citizens and still exports grain. What is her secret? One of them is sprouts! Almost everyone has eaten sprouts in their

Chinese cuisine and in Chinese restaurants. Sprouting is so simple, easy, inexpensive, and offers such bonuses of freshness and nutritional content, that it should be a common practice in inner city ghettos and other poverty areas. Research animals which show signs of malnutrition and starvation on a prolonged diet of American agribusiness produce are rejuvenated with sprouts! Malnutrition in this country could conceivably be wiped out by well-invested time and money spent in the distribution of sprouting containers and instructions to residents of tenant-farm shacks and crumbling tenements, as well as the homes of our middle class and well-to-do."

To summarize: with the regular use of sprouts, you won't have to worry about an adequate supply of amino acids and proteins; you won't have to be concerned about getting your B12 or any other vitamin or mineral; you won't have to worry about being poisoned with the chemical sprays an pesticides on your food; about calories and excessive weight; and, finally, you won't have to fear food shortages and the higher cost of food with live, fresh, organically-grown foods.

What more can we ask for? Where else can we get such a marvelous, complete, and convenient package of good nutrition at such a low cost — for *pennies*? (Dr. Wigmore says that one could eat at a cost of only 25 cents a day, if he had to.)

The wise will grasp this opportunity without delay. They will realize the importance of this subject, make a thorough study, and thereby reap the utmost benefit. Books on sprouting and on many other natural health subjects are available in most health food stores.

Growing sprouts is simplicity in itself. Nature does all the work. All you have to do is to provide the seed, water, and a suitable location for keeping the sprouts warm and moist. Filtered, purified or spring water is preferred to tap water.

Besides the method described at the beginning of this chapter, there are a number of other ways to sprout. For variety, Dr. Wigmore suggests the following simple method:

"Put a layer of wheat berries (see note below) in the bottom of a glass baking dish about an inch deep. Cover with pure water and let soak overnight. The next day, drink the water of the soaked wheat, and cover the grain with a moist towel, keeping it moist for about four days. This produces your sprouts.

"Take half of the sprouts, then cover the remainder with water, and let stand for another three days, to produce fermented sprouts. These keep well, and are delicious. You now have fresh sprouts and fermented sprouts, which keep well, and are very tasty. Both kinds of sprouts rival roast beef in protein value — in fact, are far superior to it. Sprouts do not have the many disadvantages of meat. They are fresh, living, and natural. Furthermore, sprouted seeds cost but a minute fraction of the price of meat.

"If you have a hand-operated juicer, run some of the fresh sprouts through it, and it will give you wheat milk. Add a little molasses for sweetening, if desired. There is a residue of the sprouted wheat which extrudes from the juicer. Take this residue and place it in a jar with a loose-fitting cover. Cover the residue with water, keeping the water about two inches above the level of the residue. Let it stand in a warm place, and in about one week, you will have a white mold form on the top. This white mold is wheat cheese, and is delicious."

NOTES:

WHEAT BERRIES: Wheat berries are the natural kernels of wheat. They are obtainable in health food stores, in feed stores, and by mail from companies that sell health food products. Although any type of wheat will sprout, some varieties will do so much better. Red winter wheat is one of them.

SALAD DRESSINGS: Use the recipes in this book; they will enhance the flavor of the sprouts.

SPROUTING

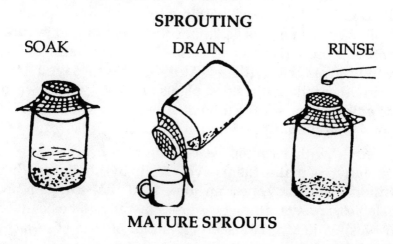

SOAK   DRAIN   RINSE

MATURE SPROUTS

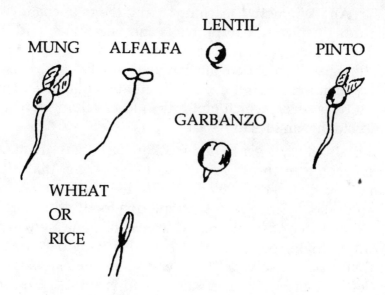

MUNG   ALFALFA   LENTIL   PINTO

GARBANZO

WHEAT
OR
RICE

A TRIBUTE TO DR. ANN WIGMORE

Dr. Ann Wigmore is a wonderful woman. From childhood in Lithuania in wartime to a position of founder and director of a famous health institute, author and lecturer, her life story sounds like a scenario. When the Nazis took all the food from her village, Ann's life was saved by a grandmother who understood plants and knew which weeds were edible. This set the tone of Ann's life. Today she is a famous "sproutarian" and humanitarian.

People with terminal cancer come to her institute, to learn how to make themselves well, by changing their nutrition from the American junk food diet to fruits and vegetables, sprouts, and wheat grass therapy. One beautiful lady was Eydie Mae Hunsberger, author of *How I Conquered Cancer Naturally*.

Dr. Ann Wigmore's teachings about the rejuvenation of cells through sprouts, natural fruits and vegetables, and the amazing wheatgrass, with its powerful chlorophyll, are truly revolutionary. Her statement that 'one can live on 25 cents per day' is not a fanciful claim, but an authentic one. That amount buys seeds, which multiply in food value. Here is a solution to the famines in Asia.

It is also the answer to this shocking fact: there are many elderly people in the U.S. with so little income that after paying their high rents, they do not have enough money left for decent food. Some turn to eating dog food! If they only had a knowledge of sprouting, which can be done anywhere, even in a single room, without soil, they would have the nutrition problem solved. They would have *Living Food at Low Cost*, full of vitamins, minerals, and enzymes. Yes, for poor people who want good nutrition for little money, sprouts are a godsend. Seeds can save them. Sprout seeds yourself and please help spread the word on sprouting.

Dr. Ann Wigmore has made it her life's work to see that the basic principles of simple and inexpensive methods of maintaining health, vitality, and greater mental alertness are available to everyone.

Now, in 1992, Dr. Wigmore is 83, still teaching and working. She is *living proof that living food maintains health, energy, and a slender body.*

She is the author of many valuable, life-enhancing and life-saving books, that should be read by all health seekers. For information, write:

Ann Wigmore Foundation
196 Commonwealth Ave.
Boston, MA 02116
Ph. (617) 267-9424

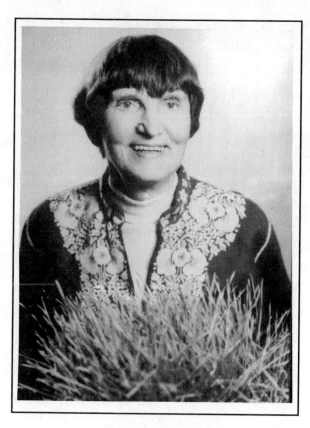

Dr. Ann Wigmore

CHAPTER VI

SUGGESTED KITCHEN EQUIPMENT

1. VEGETABLE STEAMER

This basket-like chrome or stainless steel device folds and unfolds to accommodate different quantities of vegetables. It fits into a smaller pot (for a smaller quantity of food) when properly closed.

Directions for use:

Make sure the pot you are using has a good fitting cover, then follow these easy steps:

(1) Put a small amount of water in the pot.

(2) Place the vegetables in the steamer, and

(3) Place the steamer in the pot so that only the legs are immersed in the water.

(4) Turn the heat to high, and when the steam rises,

(5) Place the lid on the pot,

(6) Turn the heat to low, and let the vegetables steam until tender.

By keeping the vegetables out of the water, the valuable nutrients and minerals are preserved, their delicate flavor retained, and very little, if any, seasoning is required.

Vegetables such as squash, cabbage, cauliflower, carrots, string beans, etc., lend themselves nicely to this softening process.

Vegetable Steamer

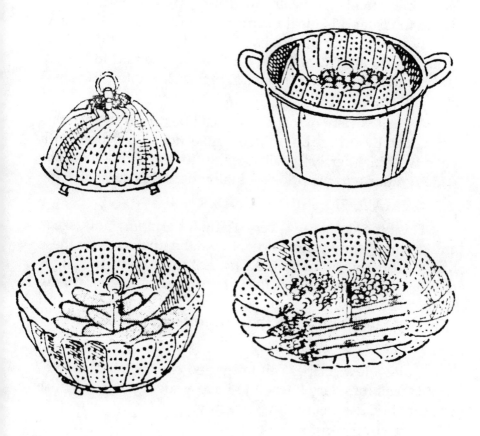

2. JUICER

Fruit juices are an excellent food. To get the most benefit from juices, they should be *fresh*. If one has a juicer, there is no problem in getting the freshly-squeezed fruit juice. Carrot juice requires another type of juicer.

3. BLENDER OR LIQUEFIER

This appliance is very handy for liquefying fruits and vegetables. It makes healthful drinks, purées and easy-to-digest foods, and is ideal for preparing foods for babies and elderly people who do not have a good set of teeth to chew with. It also affords an easy, time-saving method to liquefy and blend two or more fruits or vegetables with powdered nuts and seeds.

A great variety of tasty dishes can be prepared with this appliance. By using the printed suggestions that come with your new blender, you will be able to select those recipes which conform to the principles laid out in this manual.

4. SMALL ELECTRIC GRINDER

This little appliance is very useful for grinding nuts, seeds and grains. Many people do not take the time to chew these foods properly, or cannot, so by grinding them first, it is easier to chew and digest these hard foods. A good many recipes call for chopped or powdered nuts and seeds, and with this handy appliance, the task is greatly simplified.

5. GRATER

Quite a few recipes call for grated carrots, nutmeg, etc., so it is well for every kitchen to have a good grater. Choose one that handles easily and efficiently.

6. GARLIC PRESS

This is a small, inexpensive gadget which mashes the beads of garlic and expresses the garlic juice. This juice makes a great flavoring addition to salads and stews. On a salt-free diet, it is a good idea to use other seasoning agents along with the garlic juice — such as pepper, paprika, lemon juice, onions, herbs — to take the place of salt.

Most of these kitchen appliances are available at health food stores and in many department stores.

CHAPTER VII

MORE ORIGINAL, SALT-FREE
"HEALTHWAY" RECIPES

SECTION 1

SALAD DRESSINGS

In this section, we give you dressings that do not contain any of the harmful ingredients used in commercial dressings.

The salad dressings are first because of their great importance — both for reasons of tastiness and healthfulness. They are healthful when you use dressings made from natural ingredients, and harmful when you do not.

Here is an experience I (Bianca Leonardo) had. I seldom eat in restaurants, and on this occasion when I did so I ordered only a chopped, raw salad with a blue cheese dressing. I thought I was eating a healthful meal.

However, soon after the meal, a pain developed in my knee and then one entire leg felt paralyzed. I couldn't walk, was helped to my car, and had to go home and to bed. The salad dressing I had eaten was the only possible cause. I had never had such a problem before and have not had one since.

A brief, one-day fast, rest and simple home treatment took care of the condition quickly. This experience indicates how one ingredient can cause trouble, especially in a sensitive body. Vegetarians have more sensitive systems than other people.

In cases of arthritis, the question of salad dressings is of the utmost importance, because one wrong ingredient, such as a chemical or additive, salt or sugar, can totally interfere with the healing process.

So do not use any prepared dressings, whether in a bottle, can or package. Use only home-made dressings you prepare yourself, from natural ingredients, such as those given in this section. Please remember this. Here is one way you can "Subtract the additives" from your diet — subtracting all the harmful ingredients possible.

CARROT JUICE DRESSING

This dressing, although simple, is excellent. It consists of 2 cups of fresh carrot juice, 4 TB olive oil, and the juice of a medium-sized lemon. These three ingredients only may be used, or you may add to this mixture 1 TB granulated kelp (or 1 tsp. chili powder), and 1 tsp. garlic *powder* (not garlic *salt*). (Whenever you find "garlic salt" in recipes, use minced garlic instead.)

The carrot juice should be fresh, not canned. The canned juice has no flavor, and has harmful ingredients, as all canned goods have. If fresh carrot juice is not sold in your local health food store, you could prepare it yourself, with your own juicer. It is a marvelously healthful, inexpensive food-drink, for adults and children.

VARIATIONS:

To the above recipe, add 4 or 5 TB of cooked, chopped beets and juice.

Some of the popular herbs may be used to enhance the flavor of these salad dressings. They can be used on steamed or cooked vegetables as well as on salads.

PLAIN SALAD DRESSING

4 TBS olive oil
1 tsp. honey
2 TBS lemon juice

Mix thoroughly with an egg beater. Vary the proportions to suit your taste.

VARIATION:

Nut-Meal Dressing. Sprinkle 1 or 2 TBS of blanched almond meal (ground almonds) on top of each bowlful of salad prepared with the above salad dressing.

SPECIAL NOTE:

Many of the dressings can be varied by adding one of these: a little kelp powder; garlic powder; Brewer's Yeast; mild chili powder; dill weed powder; dash of cayenne pepper.

FRUIT JUICE DRESSING — I

2 TBS orange juice   2 TBS lemon juice
2 TBS apple, grape, or pineapple juice
1 TB honey   2 TBS homemade mayonnaise

Mix thoroughly. Naturally, for larger quantities, you will double or triple the proportions. The reason we are giving you these small quantities is that we always make our dressing fresh each time we make a salad.

FRUIT JUICE DRESSING — II

1 cup pure apple juice, unsweetened
1/2 cup olive oil
1 cup pure pineapple juice, unsweetened
1 clove garlic, minced
2 TBS sour cream or *plain* yogurt
Fresh lemon juice, to taste

The quantities of these ingredients may be adjusted to suit your taste.

FRUIT SALAD DRESSING

A simple dressing for fruit salads can be made by combining fresh orange juice with honey. Proportions may be varied to suit your taste.

FRENCH FRUIT DRESSING

4 TBS olive oil   3 TBS orange juice
3 TBS lemon juice   1TB honey

Mix ingredients with an egg beater.

WHIPPED CREAM DRESSING

4 TBS cream (or half and half)
1 TB lemon juice
1 TB honey

Whip the cream and honey together with egg beater. Slowly add lemon juice. This is a fine dressing for shredded lettuce, cole slaw, grated beets, or any fruits that are in season.

HOMEMADE MAYONNAISE DRESSING

Yolk of one egg
1 cup olive oil
2 or 3 tsps. lemon juice

Beat the yolk in a mixing bowl, adding some olive oil, drop by drop. When the mixture begins to thicken, alternately add a few drops of lemon juice and a few drops more of oil until the desired consistency is obtained. Lemon juice thins the dressing; olive oil thickens it. If more lemon juice is added, oil must also be added, as the dressing should be stiff when ready to use.

All dressings should be kept refrigerated.

VARIATION:

Add 1/2 tsp. paprika and a pinch of dry mustard powder.

AVOCADO MIX

2 cups diced, ripe avocados
1/4 cup finely chopped green onion
1 tsp. garlic powder (not garlic salt), **or**
     1 or 2 cloves minced garlic
2 TBS lemon juice
1 tsp. kelp granules

Blend or mix all ingredients well and use over salads or vegetables.

GARLIC DRESSING

Juice of 1 medium-sized lemon
3 or 4 TBS olive oil
Juice of 1 medium-sized orange
1/4 tsp. oregano
1 tsp. vinegar (aged in wood preferred)
1/4 tsp. kelp powder
2 cloves garlic, crushed

Mix all ingredients. The proportions may be varied to suit your taste.

SOUR CREAM DRESSING

1 cup sour cream
2 TBS honey
1 TB lemon juice

Whip cream and honey together until thick. Then slowly add lemon juice. Excellent for cole slaw.

Buttermilk or yogurt may be used in place of sour cream.

AVOCADO AND BUTTERMILK DRESSING

(Guacamole)

To one cup of buttermilk or yogurt, add 1/2 or 1 whole ripe avocado. Beat and blend well. Then add lemon juice, kelp powder and garlic powder to taste.

VARIATION 1:

Beat up buttermilk or yogurt with olive oil, lemon juice, a little honey and mashed avocado.

VARIATION 2:

Add 1 or 2 ripe tomatoes, skinned and chopped, to the basic recipe above.

HOMEMADE COTTAGE CHEESE AND ONION DRESSING

2 cups homemade cottage cheese (see recipe in this book)
1/2 cup or more finely-chopped green onion
1 or 2 cloves of minced garlic (optional)
Mix all ingredients and let stand for a while before using.

"HEALTHWAY" NO-SALT SEASONING

This is a mixture of kelp powder, garlic powder (not garlic salt) and Brewer's Yeast. Mix well and use in a shaker. Use on salads or vegetables or in soups. Especially delicious on toasted potatoes. (See recipe in this book.)

You can vary the proportions to suit your taste. You may use 1 cup of the yeast, 1 teaspoon of the kelp powder, and 1 teaspoon garlic powder.

This seasoning may be added to many dressings to improve the flavor. A mild chili powder may be used instead of the kelp.

HERB SEASONING

Recently we formulated a better-tasting, healthful herb seasoning with the following ingredients:
4 tablespoons Red Star Brewer's Yeast
1 tablespoon Dill Weed powder
1 or 2 teaspoons Kelp powder
2 heaping tablespoons broiled chopped onions
Fresh minced garlic to taste.

Note: In all the recipes in this book where it calls for onion and garlic powder — it would be better to use fresh broiled chopped onion and fresh minced garlic. (A garlic press is useful.)

Mix all of these well, and use as a seasoning on fresh corn on the cob, salads, steamed vegetables, and in vegetable loaves and soups.

Mixed with fresh carrot juice, it makes a delicious sauce.

The portions of the above ingredients may be varied to suit your taste. In addition, you can create a variety of flavors by adding some of the following herbs to this recipe: Basil, thyme, rosemary, marjoram, chervil, etc.

NUTRITIONAL YEAST

Nutritional or Brewer's Yeast contains good quality protein and the B Vitamins and essential amino acids. There are a number of varieties of yeast, so try different ones and choose the kind that suits your taste.

Here is an approximate analysis:

Percentage of U.S. Recommended Daily Allowances:

Protein	50%
Iron	4%
Thiamine	640%
Riboflavin	565%
Niacin	280%
Vitamin B-12	133%
Vitamin B-6	25%
Folic Acid	40%

The above is for a serving of four tablespoons.

USES OF NUTRITIONAL YEAST. As a seasoning over vegetables, in spreads, sauces, crackers, in soups and gravies. Mixed with pure bottled hot water, it makes a delicious, healthful drink. It can also be added to baby foods.

YOGURT

Yogurt is a wholesome, versatile, tasty food that can be used in various ways.

(A) Instead of sour cream or buttermilk.

(B) As a quick snack flavored with a bit of honey and a dash of cinnamon and nutmeg.

(C) Blended with fresh fruits and fresh fruit juices, it makes a refreshing drink. Use a blender for this.

(D) Flavored with minced garlic, kelp powder and herbs, it makes an unusual salad dressing.

It is better to buy plain yogurt and not the flavored variety. Flavor the yogurt yourself; then you will be sure it does not contain artificial, chemical flavoring or coloring which must be avoided by arthritis sufferers.

The Russian scientist Elie Metchnikoff discovered that the reason for the Bulgarian peasants' unusual longevity was the large amount of cultured milk, or yogurt in their diet. (With Paul Ehrlich, he won the Nobel laureate in medicine for his work on immunity on 1908.)

Culturing milk (allowing certain bacteria to grow in it) is not only a method of food preservation; cultured milk or yogurt is a wholesome food with many properties helpful to mankind.

The microorganisms* that culture dairy products make them more digestible. They can inhibit the growth of harmful bacteria that cause diarrhea, flatulence, and intestinal infection.

---

*Read the ingredients carefully on yogurt containers. For example, the widely-advertised brand "Yoplait" contains no microorganisms, but does contain aspartame (Nutrasweet) and may contain dye. On the other hand, the Mountain High brand contains active yogurt cultures (L. Bulgaricus, L. Acidophilus, L. Bifidus, and S. Thermophilus).

There are other brands in each category.

Lactobacillus acidophilus, L. bifidus, etc., are said to also help reestablish a beneficial balance in the intestines after the natural flora have been destroyed by antibiotic medication. Some studies show that cultured dairy products are anti-carcinogenic. Bacterial enzymes associated with bowel cancer have been reduced by eating *L. acidophilus.*

BACILLUS LATEROSPORUS TO THE RESCUE

A very serious condition prevalent at this time is Candidiasis, commonly called "the yeast disease." *Candida albicans* is the name of the yeast, or fungus, that creates devastating conditions of all kinds in the body.

The causes are antibiotics (which almost everyone gets from his doctor for various health problems), "The Pill," and the large amount of sugar eaten by Americans. These substances taken into the body result in an overgrowth of harmful yeast bacteria; not enough of the healthy flora remain in the body to counteract the yeast.

The Candida Research and Information Foundation states that over 80,000,000 Americans have the Candida condition. When Candida becomes systemic (permeating the entire system), it is truly serious. James B. Kless of Sacramento, California, had a crucial Candida condition. "I was suicidal," he said, "but then, fortunately, I came across a product that totally eliminated the problem—and in only eight days! It is called *Bacillus Laterosporus.* It saved my life."

Bacillus Laterosporus is its scientific name, Flora-Balance its trade name. It is not a drug, but a food product. It contains the flora that a healthy body is born with, restoring the flora to the entire system. Some persons call it "truly miraculous."

To order, call the manufacturer, Bio-Genesis, Inc., at 800–736-1991, for a source.

Tree of Life Publications can send you a report. See pages 249 and 250 of this book.

SECTION II

VEGETABLE SALADS

Again, may we remind you that salads should form the main portion of a healthful diet. If made of the right ingredients, they constitute a light, wholesome, nourishing meal in themselves. A good plan is to have a fruit bowl and a vegetable salad each day at separate meals. A fruit bowl consists of one or two fruits with one of the previously mentioned dressings or some low-fat milk or soy milk with the addition of sunflower seed meal (the seeds ground), or with blanched almonds. This makes an excellent breakfast. A green leafy vegetable or half an avocado, makes an ideal evening meal.

Salads should not be complicated with too many ingredients. The simpler they are, the easier they are to digest. They should not be too tough to chew, especially if one does not have a perfect set of teeth or does not have the time or patience to chew and chew the coarse pieces of food before swallowing.

As a rule, the finely chopped salads are easier to eat and more enjoyable. When large pieces of lettuce are served, often people will eat the mixture on top, and leave the lettuce leaves in the bowl, thus depriving themselves of the best part of the entire salad. This is true of parsley, also. It is one of the most valuable of foods nutritionally, but 95% of the parsley served is left on the plates, being considered a mere decoration. Today, there are kitchen gadgets that will do the work of chopping for you. We have a Presto "Salad Shooter"—an electric slicer-shredder.

In this book, a large number of dressings have been worked out for you so that you may choose the ones that suit your taste. Some people like their salads plain with very little dressing. Other like their salads highly seasoned. Each may have his preference.

Another factor to be considered is the temperature of the salad. It is best not to have the salad too cold, especially if the weather is cool. Often it is best to warm the salad slightly before eating, but do not cook it.

The easiest to digest and the best ingredients for salads are these: tender lettuce leaves, tomatoes, spinach, shredded cabbage, grated carrots, the various sprouts, celery, cucumbers, green onions and avocados. In areas and seasons when some of these are not available, the many kinds of sprouts should be used with any of our dressings.

The leafy vegetables, the tender roots and the sprouts supply the most essential and wholesome food contituents, which keep the blood in an alkaline condition and are, therefore, Nature's truly preventive medicine. One who partakes of this diet need not worry about vitamins, minerals, proteins and calories.

Each season of the year Nature brings forth the very wonderful miracle foods that are designed to nourish your body and maintain it in good health. But if one does not use these blessings that Nature offers, and instead depends upon the prettily-packaged, preserved and denatured foods in our supermarkets — then, sickness and disease are the results. You alone must make the choice. You are the master of your destiny. Again, "Accuse not Nature. She has done her part. Do thou but thine!"

LETTUCE AND SPINACH SALAD—I

1 head lettuce   1/2 bunch spinach

Wash the spinach leaves thoroughly and dry them with a towel. Chop the head of lettuce and the spinach, with a large, sharp knife, on a breadboard or other cutting board.

If you eat meat, do not use the same wooden board for cutting both meat and salad ingredients, because it retains bacteria. A plastic board is preferred.

Season with the olive oil and lemon juice dressing or any of the other dressings. Mix all the ingredients and warm the salad slightly, especially if the room or weather is cool or cold.

If chewing is a problem due to poor dentures, then the salad should be chopped *very fine*.

LETTUCE AND SPINACH SALAD—II

1 bunch young spinach
1/2 head lettuce
1 cucumber, chopped
2 large tomatoes

As above, wash the spinach leaves, dry and chop. Chop the lettuce and cucumber on the breadboard also, and mix all together. Add one of the "Healthway" salad dressings.

The tomatoes should be peeled, by dipping briefly into boiling water until the skin slips off. If cherry tomatoes are available, they should be used. You may wish to cut them in half. In the winter time when tomatoes are expensive and anemic, (poor in quality), then cooked and diced beets may be used instead.

Serve with toasted potatoes (see recipe) for a simple, nourishing, delicious meal.

GAZPACHO SALAD

4 small avocados	1 clove garlic
1 tsp. kelp powder	2 tsp. honey
1/2 tsp. oregano, crumbled	1/2 tsp. basil, crumbled
1 TB vinegar	1 or 2 TB lemon juice
1/3 cup olive oil	1 cup celery, chopped fine

1 cup green pepper, chopped
3 cups iceberg lettuce, shredded
1/2 cup green onion   (including tops, sliced thin)
2 cups diced tomatoes   (skin first — see previous page)

Mash garlic with kelp and honey. Add oregano, basil, vinegar and olive oil. Put in small jar with tight cover and shake to blend, then set aside to mellow at least one hour. Combine celery, green pepper, onion, tomatoes and lettuce. At serving time, toss the diced vegetables with half the dressing. Cut avocados in half (peel or not, as you desire). Arrange two halves on bed of shredded lettuce on salad plates. Spoon vegetables into center of avocados and over the sides. Add remainder of dressing. Makes 4 main course salad servings, or 8 dinner salad servings.

GOURMET GRATED CARROTS

No. 1:   Mix grated carrots with freshly-prepared almond meal. Moisten the mixture with the yogurt dressing or the homemade mayonnaise.

No. 2:   Grated carrots combine well with avocados and raisins.

BROILED PEPPERS

Green or red Bell peppers, broiled, chopped and added to vegetable salads, improve the flavor markedly.

As a general rule, it is best to combine fruits only, or vegetables only, in salads — for easier digestion. There is one exception: apples combine well with some vegetables, such as celery — as in the "Waldorf Salad" that follows.

WALDORF SALAD

Celery hearts	Raisins (optional)
Organic apples	Homemade mayonnaise
Chopped walnuts*	Lettuce leaves

Dice equal parts of the hearts of celery and organic apples. To this, add half the quantity of chopped walnuts and raisins. Mix with homemade mayonnaise dressing, and serve on crisp lettuce leaves.

*It is best to buy the walnuts in the shell, then shell and chop them yourself. They will be far fresher and natural (not chemicalized) than those you buy in packages, already shelled. You may also use almonds or filberts.

CITRUS SLAW

4 cups shredded cabbage	1/2 tsp. paprika
1/2 cup sour cream or yogurt	1/2 tsp. kelp powder
2 TBS fresh orange juice	2 TBS fresh lemon juice
1/4 tsp. garlic powder	A little honey
1/2 cup finely chopped radishes	

Place cabbage and radishes in a bowl, and mix. Combine all the remaining ingredients and pour over the cabbage and radishes.

MOCK CHICKEN SALAD

5 cups lentil sprouts
1 cup yellow pea sprouts
2 cups fresh corn (cut off the cobs)
2 green onions with tops, minced
1 TB unsalted peanut butter
2 cups celery stalks, minced
1/2 cup almond meal (almonds ground in nut grinder)
2 tsp. Brewer's Yeast
1 tsp. kelp powder
1/2 tsp. garlic powder or 1 clove garlic, minced

Put all the ingredients through a food grinder *twice*.
Serve raw as patties or croquettes.

PLAIN POTATO SALAD

4 medium potatoes	1/2 cup chopped celery
1/3 cup chopped onion	1/4 cup milk (low fat or soy)
1 tsp. kelp powder	2 TBS chopped parsley
3/4 cup mayonnaise*	

Pare potatoes and cut into quarters. Place in a medium saucepan and add 1 inch of water. Bring to boil. Cover, reduce heat and simmer until tender. While potatoes are cooking, mix celery, onion, mayonnaise, milk, kelp powder and parsley in a large bowl. When potatoes are done, drain off cooking liquid. (Save, and use in soups.) Cut potatoes into cubes while still warm. Add to dressing and mix well. Makes 4 to 8 servings.

*NOTE: *Do not use mayonnaise sold in the stores. Use the recipe in this book.*

COOKED BEETS

Beets with tops	Pure water
Vinegar and lemon juice (optional)	

We find it very handy in salad preparation to always have jars of cooked and chopped beets in the refrigerator. When the tomatoes in the markets are poor, we use beets instead.

Prepare the beets as follows: Wash 1 or 2 bunches of beets and tops thoroughly. Separate by cutting the tops from the beets, about 1" away from the joint. Cut the tops into 1" chunks. Cook all together, with the beets on the bottom. Use bottled water— sufficient water to cook the beets.

After the beets and tops are cooked, cool them. Remove skin of beets and chop them. Put all (beets, tops and juice) into jars and into the refrigerator.

You may wish to add a little vinegar and lemon juice to pickle them. They are now ready for daily use, in many ways.

COMBINATION SALAD

Make a large bed of chopped lettuce. Mix together the following: cooked onions and string beans; cooked and diced young beets; and skinned, cut up tomatoes.

Serve the mixture on the bed of lettuce and season with one of the dressings in this book, of your choice.

Variation: A handful of sprouts may be added before serving.

RAINBOW SALAD

2 large carrots
Dressing made of orange juice, lemon juice, and olive oil
1/2 - 1 cup cooked beets and juice.

Grate the carrots; add the beets and juice. Make the dressing. Place the mixture on lettuce leaves, on other salad greens, or serve alone.

This is a very colorful, tasty, and healthful salad.

SPICED BEETS

1 bunch beets (5 good-sized)
2 cloves
1/2 small onion (chopped)
1 TB vinegar
pineapple juice
apple juice

Cut off beet stems (leaving 1/2 inch-1 inch attached). Cook in water to cover, until done. Drain the beets and cool. Slip the skins off and cut off tails and remaining stems. Chop beets medium fine and place in a glass or earthenware bowl. Add the copped onion, vinegar, cloves, and enough combined pineapple juice and apple juice mixture to cover.

Place in refrigerator and let stand five days to marinate. Then proceed with "Red and Green Salad" below.

RED AND GREEN SALAD PLATE WITH SPICED BEETS

Spiced beets   1 large cucumber
Lettuce leaves   Optional: Carrot, Avocado

Arrange lettuce leaves on plates. Scoop drained, spiced beets on the leaves. Peel cucumber, cut into chunks or slices, and arrange on plates. For variation, add carrot sticks, grated carrots or avocado slices.

BEET-POTATO SALAD

1 cup cooked beets (fresh, not canned; sliced or chopped)
8 medium potatoes, cooked and sliced or chopped
1 small onion, chopped
1/2 cup sour cream or yogurt
1 cup chopped parsley
2 tsp. honey
1 tsp. kelp
1 tsp. dry mustard powder
1 TB vinegar and 1 TB fresh lemon juice
2 tsp. dill weed or caraway seed, ground

Combine honey, kelp, mustard, vinegar, lemon juice and 2 TB liquid from beets. Add sour cream or yogurt and mix well. Combine cucumbers, potatoes, onion, dill or caraway, half the parsley and beets, reserving a few slices for garnish. Pour enough sour cream dressing to moisten potato mixture and toss lightly until vegetables are well coated with dressing. Sprinkle with remaining parsley and garnish with reserved beet slices or cubes. Makes 10 to 12 servings. Serve cold or warm.

LIQUID GREEN VITAMIN SALAD

This salad is very useful for babies, children and also for adults who, for one reason or another, cannot handle any roughage or can't do any chewing due to dental trouble. It is far superior to any canned baby food and more economical. It is also good for people who are convalescing and need light, nourishing, easily-digested foods. When a patient is in bed, getting no exercise, he doesn't need heavy food. In fact, it overburdens the system and delays recovery.

The liquid salad contains an excellent supply of vitamins, minerals and enzymes. The ingredients may be varied according to the season of the year and their availability.

1 head lettuce (the greener the better),
    chopped into pieces
1/2 bunch of spinach, chopped
1/2 cup sprouts (any kind)
1 large or 2 small tomatoes, peeled
2 TBS parsley
Juice from 1 organic orange
Juice from 1/2 lemon
5 TBS olive oil
1 tsp. kelp powder
1 clove minced garlic
    or 1 tsp. garlic powder (not garlic salt)
1 TB Brewer's Yeast

Using the food blender, first liquefy the tomatoes with the fruit juices. Then liquefy the small pieces of lettuce and spinach, the parsley, and the sprouts. This will make a rich, thick, green, smooth mixture. Remove from blender, then add the other ingredients and mix well.

Here you have a rich, nourishing, healthful, liquid salad. With a baked potato or toasted potato slices (see recipes in this book), or half an avocado, it is an excellent, complete meal.

SECTION III

FRUIT SALADS

MIXED FRUIT SALAD

Cut up one ripe banana with any one or more of the fresh fruits in season, except oranges. In your nut grinder, grind either fresh almonds or hulled sunflower seeds, and mix with the fruits; then add some low-fat or soy milk.

FRUIT BOWL

1 or 2 ripe bananas	2 TBS wheat germ
1 or 2 sweet apples	1 cup low-fat or soy milk
2 TBS natural bran	

Slice the bananas. Peel and dice the apples. Mix both fruits; then add the wheat germ and bran. Pour the milk over the mixture. Blend all the ingredients. If the milk is cold, it may be slightly warmed, but not boiled. Bananas are ripe when they are speckled. Do not use before then.

BANANA AND WHEAT GERM BOWL

2 or 3 ripe, sliced bananas
3 TBS raw wheat germ
1 cup low-fat milk or almond, soy or rice milk
(see "Healthway" Beverage section). Or soy or rice milk.

Mix bananas with wheat germ; then moisten with the milk.

BANANA, SWEET APPLE BOWL

2 or 3 ripe, sliced bananas
1 or 2 organic, sweet apples, cubed
1/2 cup sunflower seed meal
    (ground, hulled sunflower seeds)
1 cup low-fat milk or almond milk

Mix bananas, apples and meal; then moisten with the milk.

APPLE AND PEAR SALAD

2 organic apples, cubed   1 cup milk (low-fat or soy)
1 cup almond meal (ground almonds)
2 Winter Nellis or other pears in season, peeled and cubed

Mix the apples, pears and almond meal. Moisten with the milk.

FRESH BERRY BOWL

1/2 cup almond meal
1/2 cup sunflower seed meal
1 cup milk (low-fat or soy)
2 cups berries in season
1 TB honey

Mix honey with the berries. Add the meal and mix. Moisten with the milk.

NOTES:

For a Waldorf salad, see the Vegetable Salad Section.

Any of the above mixtures can be added over lettuce leaves to make a luncheon salad. You may wish to reduce the amount of milk when served with lettuce.

SECTION IV

ENTREES

SAVORY NUT LOAF

3 cups finely chopped vegetables
    (onions, celery, carrots, green peppers)
1 1/2 cups almond nut milk (see Beverage Section)
1 TB savory herbs (marjoram and savory)
1 cup ground sunflower seeds
2 eggs
1 TB chopped parsley

Mix all ingredients well, put into an oiled pan and bake in a moderately hot oven for about 45 minutes.

SPINACH NUT LOAF

1 cup peanuts, (unsalted, unroasted), ground fine
1 bunch spinach, washed, dried, and cut fine
1 large onion (or 2 small ones), finely chopped
1 TB chopped parsley
1 cup sunflower meal
2 eggs, beaten

Mix all ingredients well. Put in oiled pan and bake for about 45 minutes.

PECAN LOAF

1 cup finely-chopped pecans
1 TB chopped parsley
1/2 cup sunflower seed meal
2 TBS chopped onions
2 eggs
1/2 cup peanut meal or salt-free peanut butter.

Mix all ingredients well and put into an oiled pan. Bake slowly for about 45 minutes.

VEGETABLE NUT ROAST

1/2 cup salt-free butter
1/2 cup finely chopped sunflower seeds
1 cup chopped mushrooms
3/4 cup chopped walnuts
2 large onions, finely chopped
5 eggs, beaten
1/4 cup chopped green pepper
3 cups soft whole wheat bread crumbs
3 cups grated carrots
1 1/2 cups chopped celery
Dash of each:
      basil, oregano

Melt salt-free butter in skillet, add mushrooms, onions and green pepper. Cook until tender but not browned. Combine this mixture in a large bowl with all of the remaining ingredients and mix well. Line the bottom of a 9" x 5" inch loaf pan with wax paper. Grease paper and sides of pan generously with butter. Turn the entire mixture into pan and bake at 325 degrees for 1 hour. Makes 8 servings.

SPANISH RICE

1 cup washed brown rice
1 cup tomatoes, chopped fine (fresh, not canned)
2 large onions, chopped fine
2 or 3 green peppers, chopped fine
1 tsp. kelp powder
1 tsp. garlic powder

Into a pan containing 2 cups boiling water, add all the ingredients except the seasoning. Cook until tender; then season with the kelp and garlic powder, or 1 clove minced garlic. Do not use Tamari or soy sauce because of their salt content.

STUFFED PEPPERS

6 large green peppers
3/4 cup brown rice, washed
1 qt. pure water
2 cups skinned, sliced tomatoes
1 level tsp. kelp powder
2 TBS melted, unsalted butter
1 cup chopped celery
1 cup chopped onion
1 cup whole wheat bread crumbs

Cook the rice in the water until soft, leaving very little water. Cut the peppers in halves, remove center core, wash and steam for about 10 minutes. While they are being steamed, add the celery and onion to the rice. Also add 1 cup of the tomatoes and the bread crumbs, the butter and kelp powder. Mix all the above well and stuff the pepper halves with mixture. Place in a baking dish. Pour the other cup of the skinned cut tomatoes around the peppers and bake in a moderate oven for about 30 minutes.

GARBANZO AND CARROT CROQUETTES

1 cup sprouted garbanzo beans
1/2 cup parsley, chopped
1 cup grated carrots
1 clove of garlic pressed
1/2 cup green onions
Spices
Tahini
Almond meal

Mix all the ingredients except the almond meal. Tahini is a thick sesame seed butter; add that to taste. Spices you may use are cumin, poppy seed or cayenne; add to taste.

Put all the ingredients through a hand food grinder; form into balls, and roll in the almond meal.

There is no cooking in this recipe.

SPOON SANDWICH

This is an excellent luncheon dish — a good way to use left-over chopped salad from the previous evening's dinner.

Chopped salad

Salt-free, whole-wheat bread

Any salad dressing in this chapter, or a special seasoning noted* below.

Toast as many bread slices as you need. Warm the salad slightly in a saucepan. Spread over the toast. Pour one of the salad dressings over the open-face sandwich. Eat with a fork or spoon.

This sandwich is ideal for small children and elderly people, as it requires little chewing. It is tasty and nutritious for everyone.

*NOTE

There are a number of vegetable broths and seasonings on the market, but most of them contain undesirable ingredients. It is important to make your own, using a mixture of any of the following powders: Brewer's Yeast, garlic, kelp, chili, cayenne, celery seed, caraway seed, dill weed, and natural herbs such as oregano, rosemary, thyme, etc. In any recipe in this book that calls for garlic powder, you may use minced, fresh garlic (but not garlic salt). Instead of kelp, you may substitute chili powder, but use a little less.

If you would like to have your "spoon sandwich" soft, to eat with a spoon, add pure, bottled water to one of the powdered mixtures above, and heat; pour small quantity over the "spoon sandwich."

EGGPLANT CASSEROLE

2 large onions, chopped
3/4 cup chopped celery
1 green pepper, chopped
1/4 cup olive oil
4 large skinned tomatoes, cut into chunks
1 unpeeled eggplant, in chunks
1/2 tsp. each garlic and chili powder;
    optional: 1 cup fresh mushrooms.

Sauté onions, celery, green pepper in hot oil until brown in skillet. Add remaining ingredients. Mix well. Pour into baking dish. Cover and cook 20-30 minutes at 350 degrees.

VEGETABLE PROTEIN PATTIES

1/4 c. chopped raw almonds
1 c. cooked brown rice
1 c. cooked lentils
1 TB sodium-reduced soy sauce
1 tsp. dried oregano, crushed
3/4 tsp. dried thyme, crushed
1/4 tsp. freshly ground black pepper
1/8 tsp. cayenne pepper, or to taste
1/2 cup grated carrot
1 cup uncooked oatmeal

Preheat oven to 350° F. Toast almonds in oven for about 8 minutes or until a deep golden brown; do not burn. Set aside.

Combine rice, lentils, soy sauce, oregano, thyme, black pepper and cayenne in a food processor and mix until smooth. Place mixture in a bowl and add grated carrot, oatmeal and toasted almonds; mix thoroughly. Form mixture into 8 quarter-cup patties. Spray a skillet with non-stick vegetable coating and heat until a drop of water bounces on the surface before evaporating. Place patties in skillet and cook until lightly browned on both sides.

WALNUT PATTIES

1 cup ground walnuts
1 cup dried whole wheat bread crumbs
1 cup almond meal
1 grated carrot, medium
1 onion chopped fine, medium
2 eggs, beaten
2 cups strained fresh tomato pulp

Mix all of the above ingredients excepting the tomato pulp and form into small patties. Cover with the tomato pulp and bake for 20 minutes.

BEANS AND LEGUMES

Beans are a good source of protein; soybeans are the highest. To get all the essential amino acids, combine beans with whole grains, or nuts and seeds.

Preparation: Wash beans in cold water and pick out the poor ones. Soak beans from 8 to 10 hours, or overnight. (Lentils and peas do not require soaking.) Place beans in large pan made of one of the heavy materials (stainless steel, baked enamel, earthenware, etc.) Use the water the beans were soaking in, and add more, to cover beans. The usual amount is 3 to 4 cups water to 1 cup dried beans. Seasoning is added during the last 20 minutes.

EASY BAKED BEANS

1 medium onion, chopped
2 cups cooked kidney or pinto beans
1/2 cup vegetable stock
1 cup tomato sauce
1 or 2 cloves garlic, chopped
1 to 2 tsp. chili powder, or 1 cup stewed tomatoes

Sauté garlic and onion in stock until tender. Mix with remaining ingredients and place in baking pan. Cover and bake in 350°F. oven 1-2 hours. Serve warm. Makes 4 to 6 servings. Double ingredients for a larger quantity, to freeze for later meals.

SECTION V

VEGETABLES

Vegetables are insufficiently appreciated. They all have basic food elements the body needs for health. Preparation is important, also.

CARROTS are an excellent source of Vitamin A.* Vitamin A helps maintain normal vision in dim light, protects against infection, and aids in developing normal bones and teeth.

*One medium carrot provides 330% of the U.S. Recommended Daily Allowance (RDA).

The carrot is low in sodium, and low in calories (only 25 calories per serving). The raw carrot (whole, grated, or in freshly-made carrot juice) is more valuable than the cooked. We use both raw carrots and the juice, but, of course, the former also gives you fiber, while with juice, the fiber is discarded. (Give it to your pets, if any, mixed with their food, so it is *not* wasted.)

Carrots are a major dietary source of beta-carotene, now known to play a key role in the body's resistance to cancer. If you replace your meat dishes with carrots and other vegetables, you have taken a major step against the development of cancer.

MASHED CARROT

6 medium to large carrots
Seasoning: pepper or health type; (no salt)
1/4 - 1/2 cup milk (low-fat or soy)
2 - 3 TBS unsalted butter or soy margarine

Wash and scrape the carrots and cook them in a small amount of boiling water. Drain, reserving the liquid for a soup base. Mash the carrots as you would potatoes, adding just enough milk to make them fluffy. Season, place into a serving dish, and top with the unsalted butter or soy margarine.

Preparation time: 20 minutes; serves 4 to 6. This is a very simple but unusual, and wholesome dish.

CARROT LOAF

2 cups grated carrots
2 cups soft bread cubes
2 cups diced, fresh tomatoes
2 small onions, minced

3 eggs, beaten
1 tsp. seasoning of your
    choice (not salt)
Pepper, if desired to taste

Preheat oven to 350°. Mix all ingredients together in a large mixing bown and bake, uncovered, in casserole for 1 hour, or until center is firm.

Most vegetables, such as cabbage, cauliflower, broccoli, squash, etc., can be quickly and easily steamed.

They may be eaten with a salad, with avocado, unsalted butter, or with one of the dressings given in this chapter.

STEAMED BROCCOLI

Wash and dry the stems and flowers. Cut the flowers off and lay aside. Cut off the tough outside covering of the stem, and discard. Then divide the stems into chunks about one inch long. Using the vegetable steamer described in our "Kitchen Equipment" chapter, steam the stem sections a little; before they are well done, add the broccoli flowers and steam all until tender.

The steamed broccoli may be eaten alone, with half an avocado, or with a salad, using any one of the dressings in this chapter.

STEAMED CAULIFLOWER

Wash and dry the cauliflower and separate the buds. Steam until tender. This requires very little cooking.

This dish may be eaten alone, with or without any one of the dressings in this book, or with a salad or avocado.

STEAMED ZUCCHINI SQUASH

3 large onions   2 lbs young, tender Zucchini squash
2 TBS olive oil

Chop the onions fine, and sauté in olive oil in a frying pan until brown. Wash the squash well and cut off both ends (one end will be tough; both ends may have bits of sand in them). Cut squash into 1 1/2" chunks; place in steamer and steam until squash is tender and mashes easily with a fork or masher. After mashing, add the sautéed onions, mix well and serve.

STEAMED SUMMER SQUASH

Follow the same recipe as for Steamed Zucchini Squash.

STEAMED CABBAGE

Cut a head of cabbage into four, six, or eight sections. Place these into your steamer and cook until tender.

Cabbage may be eaten alone with a little *unsalted* sweet butter, or with avocado, or with a salad.

GOURMET RED CABBAGE

Take one red cabbage, cut in quarters and steam in your vegetable steamer. Now serve with one of the following natural sauces and dressings:

(1)   Buttermilk and lemon juice; serve over warm cabbage.

(2)   Mashed avocado + buttermilk + lemon juice; + seasoning (not salt); pour over the cabbage quarter; top with paprika. Colorful as well as delicious.

(3)   Serve lemon wedges with the cabbage quarter, to be squeezed over the vegetable by the diner.

(4)   Pour diluted cider vinegar over hot red cabbage.

(5)   Serve caraway seed + sunflower seeds, ground in your nut grinder + buttermilk.

This tasty and attractive vegetable, with one of these delicious dressings, can be a meal in itself. It is very economical, also.

VARIATION: Green cabbage can be used the same way.

MUSHROOM LOAF

3 cups chopped mushrooms, fresh
Sweet butter or soy margarine
2 cups chopped onions
Low-fat milk or soy or rice milk
1/2 cup sunflower seed meal
1/2 cup almond meal
1/2 tsp. kelp powder
1 garlic clove, minced or
1/2 tsp. garlic powder (not garlic salt)

Sauté the mushrooms and onions in the sweet butter. Add the sunflower and almond meal. Season with the kelp and garlic (minced or powder). Moisten with a little milk. Mix well and turn into a baking dish with a cover. Bake for 25 minutes at 300 degrees.

VEGETABLES OVER BROWN RICE

Choose any combination of carrots, broccoli, cauliflower, red cabbage, green peppers, scallions, tomatoes, mushrooms, cilantro (all cut small). You may add unsalted cashew halves. Sauté in 1 TB water, 1 TB minced garlic, and 1 TB olive oil. When soft, serve over brown rice, which is cooking at the same time.

POTATOES

(Toasted; Baked — see Chapter IV.)

GREEN BEANS LYONNAISE

1 tsp. garlic powder or minced garlic
2 lbs. green beans
3 tsp. sweet, unsalted butter
1/2 tsp. kelp powder
1 cup minced onions

Cook beans in as little water as possible, then drain any excess water. Or use a steamer.

Melt butter in a skillet; add onions and cook until browned. Mix in kelp and garlic, toss with beans.

HERBED SUMMER SQUASH CASSEROLE

2 pounds summer squash, sliced
1 onion, thinly sliced
2 tomatoes, peeled and chopped
1/2 tsp. kelp powder
1/2 tsp. garlic powder
1/2 tsp. basil
1/2 tsp. oregano
3 TBS unsalted butter

Combine squash, tomatoes and onion in a greased casserole, layering or mixing the vegetables according to personal preference. Sprinkle with kelp, dill weed, basil and oregano. Dot with unsalted butter. Bake at 350 degrees, 30 - 40 minutes, or until squash is tender.

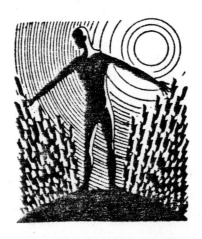

"Accuse not Nature, she hath done her part;
Do thou but thine!"

—John Milton

SECTION VI

SOUPS and STEWS

LIMA BEAN STEW

1/2 lb. large lima beans
Distilled water
3 onions
2 cups diced celery
2 bay leaves
1 clove garlic, chopped fine
4 large tomatoes, skinned

Soak the lima beans in hot boiled water for several hours. The skins will then come off easily when pressed. Discard the skins. Cook the onions and celery in a large pot with just enough water to cover. Add the skinned lima beans and the water in which they were soaked. Next, add the bay leaves and garlic. Cook until the limas are tender, then add the tomatoes. Cook a few minutes more until the tomatoes are done.

POTATO SOUP

2 large onions, chopped fine
4 large potatoes, diced
4 cups water
1 cup chopped parsley
1 cup chopped celery stalks
Kelp powder
Garlic powder
Brewer's Yeast

Cook the onions in very little water in a large pot, until well done. Then add the potatoes, water, parsley and celery. Cook until all the vegetables are tender. Season with kelp powder, garlic powder and Brewer's Yeast.

CABBAGE AND CARROT STEW

3 large onions
3 cups distilled water
3 eggs
1 bunch carrots, diced
1 small cabbage, or 1/2 large cabbage, chopped
Dash of cayenne pepper
1/2 avocado

Chop and boil the onions in the water in a large pot. When done, add the chopped cabbage and diced carrots. (If necessary, add a little more water.) Cook until both are tender, then slightly beat the eggs and add to the mixture. Cook the stew for another minute or two until the eggs are set. Season with the dash of cayenne, and serve with half an avocado.

CARROT-PEAS-AND-ONION STEW

1 bunch carrots
2 large onions
2 cups fresh peas, shelled
1 avocado (optional)

Scrape and grate the carrots. Chop and cook the onions in as little water as possible. When done, add the carrots and cook until slightly tender. Add the peas and cook until tender. Serve with half an avocado, if available.

Optional: Use carrot juice dressing on top of this delicious stew.

Note: If fresh peas are not in season you may use frozen peas, but not canned. Make sure the frozen peas are not seasoned with salt, sugar, or a sauce.

BEAN POT

1 lb. navy beans
6 cups water
2 cups bean liquid
1/2 cup molasses
2 tsp. dry mustard
1/2 cup honey
1 large onion, chopped

Soak beans in heated water for at least 6 hours. Cook onion until well done. Add soaked beans to cooked onions, and cook until beans are tender. Then add the other ingredients.

BORSCHT

3 medium beets
1 cup finely chopped carrots
5 cups water
1 cup finely shredded cabbage
1 to 2 TBS lemon juice
2 TBS minced onion
Kelp and garlic powder
Yogurt or sour cream

Boil beets 15 minutes in enough water to cover. Drain, remove skins and dice. Place beets, carrots and water in a saucepan. Cook for 20 minutes, covered. Add cabbage, lemon juice and onion, Heat to boiling; reduce heat and simmer 20 minutes, covered. Serve hot or cold. Garnish each bowl with a tablespoon of sour cream or yogurt.

SPLIT PEA SOUP

1/2 lb. split peas
2 large, finely chopped onions
2 cups finely chopped celery stalks
2 cups grated carrots
1 cup chopped parsley
1 large potato, diced
6 cups water

Wash and soak the split peas in very hot water for an hour. Cook the finely chopped onions in very little water in a large pot until they are well done. Then add all the above ingredients, and cook until they are tender. Season with kelp powder, garlic powder and Brewer's Yeast.

VEGETABLE SOUP

1 cup grated carrots
2 cups chopped onions
1 cup green peppers, finely chopped
1 cup parsnips
1 cup finely chopped celery
1 cup shelled peas
1 lb. tomatoes
1/2 cup chopped parsley
1/2 pound string beans, cut in small pieces
1 tsp. kelp powder
1 tsp. garlic powder
1 tsp. Brewer's Yeast

Mix and cook all the above except the tomatoes, slowly until they are tender. Then add the tomatoes and simmer until they are done. Season with kelp powder, garlic powder and Brewer's Yeast.

RICH LENTIL SOUP

1 cup lentils
1 cup diced celery
1 1/2 quarts distilled water
5 large onions
4 large tomatoes, peeled and quartered
1 cup diced carrots
2 TBS olive oil
1 tsp. kelp powder
1/2 cup chopped parsley
1 tsp. garlic powder

First look through the lentils for foreign matter that may possibly be there. Wash the lentils and cover with hot water. Soak for a few hours. Dice four of the onions and sauté them in olive oil until brown. Chop one onion and cook until tender in remaining water in a large pot. Add the diced carrots and celery and the soaked lentils. Cook until the carrots and lentils are soft and tender. Remove the skin of the tomatoes by immersing them in boiling water for a minute or two. Add the tomatoes and parsley to the lentils and cook for five minutes. Add the sautéed onions and serve. Season with kelp and garlic powder.

BARLEY SOUP

1 cup whole barley
4 cups water
1 finely chopped onion
1/2 cup chopped celery stalk
1 TB chopped parsley
2 cups almond milk

Cook the barley and onions in the water until the barley is very soft. Then add the vegetables and boil for another 20 minutes.

This soup may be seasoned with any of the seasonings in this book.

VEGETABLE STOCK

To create your own vegetarian soups, you will need a supply of vegetable stock. We find that vegetable bullion cubes (when you can find them) are very salty, and insufficient in quantity.

Few things can improve the flavor of your cooking as quickly and easily as a vegetable stock, which is made by simmering savory ingredients in water until their flavors transfer to the liquid. The stock keeps well and will last up to nine months in the freezer. This recipe makes ten cups.

3 stalks celery, with leaves	2 yellow onions
1 whole leek, with tops	(peels on; quartered)
1 summer squash	12 cups pure water
3 carrots	4 peppercorns
3 garlic cloves	2 bay leaves
(not peeled, but crushed)	1/4 teaspoon thyme
1 bunch parsley (stems only)	

Cut the celery, leek, squash, and carrots into 2-inch chunks. Put them and the rest of the ingredients into a 6-quart stockpot. Bring to a boil, then reduce to a simmer. Skim off and discard any sediment that floats to the surface. Cover and cook for 35-40 minutes. The longer it is cooked, the stronger the flavor. Discard the vegetables. (Or—if you have a pet, you can mix with his food.) Strain the broth through a fine sieve or cheesecloth.

SECTION VII

BREADS and CAKES

WHOLE WHEAT BREAD

3 1/2 cups whole wheat flour (about 1 pound)
1 1/2 cups almond milk, low fat milk, or soy milk
2 TBS honey
1/2 cake yeast
2 TBS finely chopped onions

Slightly heat the milk with the honey. When lukewarm, add the yeast, first mixing it into a paste with a little milk. Add the flour and chopped onions. Knead well and let it double in volume. Again knead it thoroughly. Put into oiled pans, leaving sufficient room for it to rise. Bake in moderately hot oven (350 degrees) for about 50 minutes.

WHOLE WHEAT GEMS

2 cups almond nut milk or 2 cups sour milk
3 cups whole wheat flour (or enough to make a batter)
1 egg
2 TBS very finely chopped onion

Thoroughly mix the nut milk or the sour milk with the yolk of the egg and the onion. Then add the flour a little at a time to retain as much air as possible in the mixture. Then mix in the well-beaten white of the egg. Put into gem irons which have been heated and oiled. Bake for about 45 minutes.

CARROT CAKE

1 3/4 cups almonds*
3 eggs, separated
1 1/4 cups honey
1/2 cup whole wheat flour
Grated rind and juice of 1 organic lemon ‡
3 cups coarsely grated raw carrots**
     * Measure before putting thru nut grinder
   ** Measure after grating

Mix all ingredients well, except the egg whites. Beat the egg whites until stiff and fold into the mixture. Butter two small pans or one 9" pan, and line with buttered waxed paper, or muffin tins. Bake at 300 degrees until light brown, then let cool slowly in oven 30 minutes longer.

‡ If you do not have an organic lemon, use only the juice, not the rind. Use a small size lemon, or half of a large one.

UNFIRED FRUIT CAKE

1 cup almond meal (use blanched almonds)
1/2 tsp. cinnamon
1 cup pitted dates, finely minced
1 cup black figs, finely minced
1 large, juicy, organic apple, grated

Mix all ingredients thoroughly by running them through a food chopper or blender. If necessary, add a little fresh fruit juice to make a thick paste. Press into a loaf pan. Freeze in freezer. Slice before serving.

CAROB-APPLE BARS

1/2 cup honey
2 TBS unsalted butter
1 cup shredded peeled apple
2 tsp. vanilla
1/2 cup whole wheat flour
1 egg, lightly beaten
1/2 cup chopped walnuts
2 cups oats
3/4 cup carob powder

Combine honey, apple, butter in a bowl. Blend well. Stir in vanilla, flour, egg, walnuts, oats and carob powder. Mix well. Let stand at least ten minutes for the oats to absorb the moisture. Turn into lightly greased 8 or 9-inch square pan. Bake at 375 degrees for 25 minutes. Cut into bars when cool. Makes 18 bars.

HONEY COCONUT MACAROONS

2 cups almond meal
1/2 cup honey
1 cup hot water
1 cup shredded coconut
2 cups whole wheat flour

Mix thoroughly the almond meal, honey and hot water. Then stir in the shredded coconut and flour. Put into convenient shapes on a well-oiled pan and bake in a moderately hot oven for about 1/2 hour.

ALMOND CAKE with PEACHES and CREAM

1 cup almonds
3/4 cups honey
6 eggs, separated
1/2 tsp. cinnamon
1/2 cup sunflower seed meal
1 organic lemon
6 kernels of peach or prune pits

Grease a 10" x 6" or 11" x 7" shallow pan with sweet butter or soy butter (at room temperature), or olive oil. Line with waxed paper and grease again.

With electric grinder, grind almonds and fruit kernel pits. Beat egg whites until soft peaks form. Add honey and beat until stiff. Beat egg yolks with grated lemon peel and juice and pour over egg whites. Sprinkle ground almonds and ground sunflower seeds over mixture and blend well. Turn into prepared pan and bake at 250 degrees for 40 to 50 minutes. Cool before removing from pan. Peel off waxed paper and store in refrigerator. Serve with fresh or frozen sliced peaches and cream.

This cake has no flour, which is remarkable. Flour, in general, is not a healthful ingredient. It is far removed from the original, natural cereal. The less flour one uses, the better.

RAISIN BRAN MUFFINS

2 cups plain bran
2 cups whole wheat flour
1 cup finely chopped almonds
1/2 cup raisins
1 egg; 1/2 cup honey
1 TB melted sweet butter
1 1/2 cups low-fat milk or buttermilk

Mix all the ingredients well and pour into well-buttered muffin pan, or use muffin paper cups. Bake in moderate oven. Let muffins cool before removing from pan.

The following article appeared in 'The Los Angeles Times, on October 22, 1970. It speaks for itself:

NUTRITIONISTS'S CHARGE —

"ENRICHED BREAD PUT ON PAR WITH SAWDUST"

A nutritionist told the National Academy of Sciences that the "enriched" bread most Americans eat has about the same nutritional value as sawdust.

Dr. Roger J. Williams said that tended to prove the food industry has done nothing to assist a public nutritional problem, and may even be regressing.

The charge was made in a paper at the fall meeting of the academy at Rice University. Dr. Williams is associated with the Clayton Foundation Biochemical Institute, University of Texas in Austin.

"In spite of improved infant feeding which has been made evident by some increase in stature, it has seemed to the writer that the food industries in general tend to remain static (or even regressive) with respect to providing the public with better and better food, " he wrote.

He reported a test made with the "enriched" bread now used by most Americans. Sixty-four rats of four different strains were given the commercial bread. Matched groups were given the same bread supplemented along the lines science shows is needed . . . .

After two weeks, the strains getting the improved bread gained from 4.8 to 9.5 times as much weight as those on "enriched" bread. After 90 days, two-thirds of those on the commercial bread were dead of malnutrition. The rats on the supplemented bread were doing well.

SECTION VIII

CEREALS and BREAKFAST RECIPES

WHOLE WHEAT CEREAL

3 eggs
1 cup low-fat milk or soy milk
4 TBS wheat germ

Beat the eggs well with the milk. Add the wheat germ and mix well. Cook in a well-oiled pan until the eggs are done. Be careful not to overcook. Remove from the heat as soon as the mixture gets firm.

ONION OMELET

2 large onions, finely chopped
3 eggs
1 cup low-fat milk or soy milk

Sauté the onions until browned. Beat eggs with the milk. Grease the pan with either olive oil or unsalted butter. Mix all the ingredients and cook until the mixture becomes semi-solid, while stirring with a fork.

VARIATION: TOMATO and ONION OMELET

Cut tomatoes into small pieces. Chop onions fine. Cook onions in *unsalted* butter in saucepan until soft. Add cut-up tomatoes and cook a few minutes more. Prepare the omelet and when ready to fold, add the onions and tomatoes.

HEALTH BREAKFAST NO. 1

1 lb. prunes — uncooked, unprocessed
Water (pure)

Soak the prunes in enough water to completely cover them, in a bowl or pot, for 48 hours. They will become plump and soft. Transfer to a mason jar and keep in the refrigerator, using them as needed.

1 dozen prunes, prepared as above
3 TBS plain bran flakes
2 TBS wheat germ
2 cups low-fat milk or soy milk
1/2 cup sunflower meal
1/2 cup almond meal

For one serving, put the prunes into a dish. Then add the other ingredients and mix well. This makes a nourishing, healthful, delicious breakfast, or substantial dessert after a light meal.

HEALTH BREAKFAST NO. 2

2 ripe bananas, sliced
Low-fat milk or soy milk
One dozen soaked prunes (see previous recipe)

Mix the bananas, prunes and milk. The proportions may be varied to suit your taste.

Variation: Almond and sunflower seed meal may be added to this dish, also.

POTATO PANCAKES

5 potatoes
1/2 cup low-fat milk or soy milk
1 egg, beaten
1 onion
1/2 tsp. kelp powder
1/2 cup wheat germ
1/2 cup plain bran flakes
Buttermilk or plain yogurt

Parboil the potatoes in the skins for about 10 minutes. Remove the skins and chop the potatoes fine. Add the milk, egg, onion, kelp powder, wheat germ and bran flakes. Mix well into a smooth batter. Shape into patties and bake in a buttered pan until brown. Serve with the buttermilk or plain yogurt.

GRANOLA

6 cups rolled oats
1 1/2 cups sunflower seed meal
1 1/2 cups sesame seeds
1 1/2 cups almond meal
1/2 cup raisins
1 1/2 cups wheat germ
1/2 cup honey
1/2 cup low-fat milk or soy milk
1/2 tsp. cinnamon

Mix all ingredients well. Then place the mixture in a large, flat, open pan and broil for about 15-20 minutes, stirring the mixture at frequent intervals. Be sure not to burn it. Cool, then place in glass jars and store in refrigerator. Serve with sliced raw fruit in season and moisten with low-fat or soy milk.

SECTION IX

BEVERAGES

WATER is an important component of the human body. It is being used and lost continually through the lungs, skins, and other organs of elimination. It is highly essential that it be replenished by the food we eat and the liquids we drink. If you will refer to the *Basic Diet* suggested at the beginning of this manual, you will note that large percentages of fresh fruits and fresh vegetables are included. These fresh foods contain a great deal of pure, organic water which the body needs and uses for all its functions.

When the diet consists of such a good supply of watery foods, there is little need for drinking water. However, when any water is needed for drinking or cooking, it should be of good quality. The water coming from our faucets is anything but that. It is loaded with strong chemicals that do not belong in the body and can cause trouble, especially in cases of arthritis. It is therefore advisable to use bottled water which is distilled, or pure, spring water, free from added chemicals.

In some of our cities, the public water supply is fluoridated. This is bad for arthritis, so the use of bottled or filtered water is advisable. There are a number of inexpensive water filtering appliances on the market. It would be a good precaution to purchase and use one of these appliances.

A water distiller is more expensive, but is more thorough in its purifying process.

"HEALTHWAY" BEVERAGES

(In preparing any of these drinks, use bottled, filtered, or distilled water whenever possible.)

COFFEE: To round out the diet, most of us will want a hot drink. As is well known, coffee, with its ingredient caffeine, is harmful.

Instant coffee, when taken with white sugar, is a potent cause of arthritis and should be strictly avoided. In the process of making instant coffee, the companies use certain chemicals which have an adverse effect in cases of arthritis.

If you must have coffee, use the *regular ground coffee* with honey as a sweetener. Also, use less coffee by combining it with any of the coffee substitutes in this chapter.

The coffee break seems like a harmless, pleasant pastime — but it is anything but harmless. If people knew how coffee upsets the normal functions of the body, and in that way brings on many ill effects, they would think twice before using this habit-forming drink.

Coffee is a stimulant that "picks you up," and then "lets you down." It stimulates the secretions of the acid gastric juices, which irritates the lining of the stomach and helps to cause ulcers.

Many tests have shown that coffee is a definite cause of disorders of the thyroid gland—one of the most important glands of the body, because it regulates many of the bodily functions. It regulates the way food is broken down and built into cells. It controls the way the body uses the minerals in our foods. It influences the growth of the body. It regulates the reproductive functions. It influences our emotions, our behavior and our personalities.

So you can see how one unnatural food or beverage can upset the delicate balance of the bodily functions, and thus bring on many ailments.

You should try to give up the use of coffee. If you feel you must have it, then use a small amount mixed with any one of the following recommended coffee substitutes. But make sure you never use it with sugar added, or combine it with cake, pie, or other desserts made with sugar. Also, as stated, use the regular grind instead of the instant coffee.

In place of coffee, we use and recommend the following beverages:

ROASTED DANDELION ROOT and GRAIN BEVERAGE: This beverage is a rich, coffee-like blend of roasted grains and roasted dandelion roots, sweetened with carob and spices. Served with a little milk, or soy milk, it makes a most delicious, satisfying drink. It will help you give up coffee. This herbal beverage is sold in most health food stores.

Check such stores for other, similar products. One is called "Pero." Its ingredients are: malted barley, barley, chicory and rye. Another is Amazake, a very delicious creamy rice drink, naturally sweet.

SOYBEAN COFFEE: This is a cereal coffee made by roasting soybeans, then grinding them, and using as one would use coffee. By sweetening with honey and adding low-fat milk, or soy milk, you will have a pleasant coffee substitute.

CEREAL COFFEES: All of these are tasty and healthful coffee substitutes. They are drinks that "pick you up, but don't let you down."

(1) This beverage is made of roasted barley, chicory and molasses. It can be used with honey and low-fat milk, almond milk or soy milk. To make it, you roast some barley, grind it, mix it with chicory and molasses.

(2) Use chicory alone, with water, low-fat milk (or soy or rice milk) and honey.

(3) Use roasted carob powder, water, low-fat milk (or soy or rice milk) and honey.

(4) Use equal parts of chicory and carob powder; water, low-fat milk (or soy or rice milk) and honey.

Prepare as you do coffee.

OTHER "HEALTHWAY" BEVERAGES

ALMOND MILK: Grind into a fine powder 1 cup of blanched and dried almonds. Add hot (bottled) water to the meal, and beat thoroughly or blend. A blender is preferred, but if you do not have one, use an egg beater. Then add a little honey or fresh fruit juice. The amount of hot water and fruit juice will depend upon the consistency you want the almond milk to be. Almond milk may be used by those who are allergic to cow's milk, including babies. It can be used in many recipes and over fruit salads or fruit bowls.

FRUIT JUICES help to round out a well balanced diet, but caution should be used when they are added to the basic diet because some of the ready-prepared juices contain chemical preservatives and refined sugar.

Fresh, home-made organic fruit juices are the best, but if they are not available, then the ready-made juices should be added one at a time, and a record kept in a notebook for this purpose. If pain occurs, you should consult the notations in your notebook to see which of the juices you used; then stop using the offending items.

Bottled apple juice labeled "Pure Apple Juice — No Sugar Added" is one of the safer ones. As for the others, you will have to test them to make sure they do not cause any unwanted reaction.

FRESH ORANGE JUICE: Made of ripe, organic oranges, this is delicious and good for you. But if the oranges are embalmed or sour, don't use them. *VARIATION:* To 1/2 cup boiling (bottled) water, add 1/2 cup freshly squeezed orange juice. Heat slightly but do not boil. Add honey to the desired sweetness.

PINEAPPLE and APPLE JUICE DRINK: These two juices, mixed half and half, make a tasty drink that can be used warm or cold.

FRESH CARROT JUICE: The freshly prepared juice of the carrot is a marvelous food and drink. It is abundantly rich with Nature's finest and purest nutrients, is very delicious, and one of great value for young and old. It is of special benefit for anyone suffering with arthritis. In the beginning, when the arthritis sufferer is changing from the ordinary, disease-producing diet to the natural-hygienic diet, carrot juice should be consumed liberally. The important point to remember is to have it fresh. You can buy it in many health food stores; it should be shaken frequently so that the calcium sediment becomes mixed throughout the bottle. Freshness is important; it is best to invest in your own juicer and consume the carrot juice immediately after preparing.

Remember that carrot juice is a food. Do not drink it down fast, as you would water. Sip it slowly and salivate it before swallowing. The enzymes in the saliva need to work on it before it is swallowed.

BLACKSTRAP MOLASSES DRINK: To three cups of water, add three tablespoons of molasses. Boil and add low-fat milk, or soy milk. Try the various brands of molasses to find the taste you like best, but make sure the product is *not* treated with sulphur. Read the labels.

HOT WATER, MILK AND HONEY DRINK: Boil water, add low-fat milk or soy milk, and honey. This makes a fine, mild, soothing drink.

HERBAL TEAS: At your health food store you will find a wide assortment of natural herb teas, such as chamomile, comfrey, peppermint and many others. These may be used with honey and a little lemon juice, or just plain. *Chamomile* is especially valuable. Just one ounce of chamomile flowers mixed with a pint of boiling water, taken hot or cold, provides a *natural*, safe, soothing and delicious *sedative*. It soothes the nerves, relaxes the body, helps stomach problems and is sleep-inducing.

Try various kinds of herbal teas. You will find some which are very delicious and satisfying. Select your favorites and use only herbal teas.

BLACK and GREEN TEAS

Most teas are artificially colored. True, the green tea is not colored, but all these teas contain tannin, or tannic acid, which has harmful effects on the body. (This acid is used to tan leather.) It is better to use herbal teas, which have a soothing effect on the system.

SECTION X

DESSERTS and CONFECTIONS

IMPORTANT INFORMATION ON DESSERTS

Dried fruit and nut confections should take the place of ordinary candy, which contains sugar, artificial coloring, artificial flavoring, chemical additives and preservatives — all of which cause much trouble in the body.

Those suffering with arthritis should strictly avoid these artificial confections, and instead use those made of wholesome, natural ingredients.

In choosing your nuts, seeds and dried fruits, be careful to get good quality. The nuts should be fresh and the dried fruit should not be bleached and processed with preservatives.

The following are some good and easy-to-make recipes:

STUFFED DATES

Remove the pit by opening the side of the date with a knife. Insert half of a shelled pecan, or a blanched almond.

STUFFED PRUNES

Remove the pit of the prune and insert a half walnut, pecan, or blanched almond.

STUFFED FIGS

Cut open one side of the fig and stuff a blanched almond between the two halves. Then close the opening.

NUTS — NUT MEAL — NUT MILK

Nuts and seeds are Nature's most concentrated foods. They are very high in nutritive value, especially protein.

The protein in nuts and seeds is far superior to animal protein, for at least three good reasons. Nuts and seeds:

1. Can be eaten raw. Cooking destroys the vitamins and enzymes.

2. They are much easier to digest than meat.

3. They are not as perishable and, if organic, are not treated with chemicals that aggravate arthritis symptoms.

One of the best nuts is the almond, and of the seeds, the sunflower seed.

Those who have a good set of teeth may eat them whole. But if the teeth are in poor shape, or the person has dentures, then the nuts and seeds are better ground into a meal.

Nut meal may be used for baking purposes, such as nut loaves, and for making various kinds of fruit and nut confections.

Nut meal is also excellent to sprinkle over fruit and vegetable salads. This gives added protein to a salad, making it a complete dish, and nuts blend well with fruits and vegetables. This is a good combination.

With a food blender, nut meal can be made into a nut milk by adding pure water and a little honey.

For children and adults who are allergic to cow's milk, the nut milk serves very well. It has no harmful side effects, as cow's milk often has. It is ideal for vegetarian children.

THE CHOCOLATE PROBLEM SOLVED

Chocolate is a very popular confection. By definition, chocolate is a combination of cocoa with white sugar. Many students of nutrition have studied the effects of chocolate on the human body and have come to the conclusion that this confection is responsible for a number of harmful allergic reactions on the body — such as skin eruptions, vomiting, etc. Chocolate is addictive, fattening, and injurious to the teeth.

In cases of arthritis, it very often interferes with recovery, and for that reason you should avoid using it. Fortunately, there is an excellent substitute for chocolate, and that is CAROB POWDER. This natural food product is made from the fruit of the carob tree which grows in many subtropical areas. Since Biblical times, the carob fruit has been used as food, and is also known as St. John's Bread.

When this carob powder is combined with honey, it makes a delicious confection that looks and tastes very much like chocolate, and—best of all—may be eaten without fear of any unpleasant allergic reactions.

When you purchase carob powder, be sure it contains NO SUGAR.

HOT CAROB FUDGE SUNDAE SAUCE

1 cup honey
1 cup milk (low fat, soy or rice)
1 cup roasted carob powder

Combine carob powder with the milk in the top of a double boiler. When smooth, add the honey. Cook until soft ball stage is reached. This may take half an hour.

Pour over scoop of ice cream, for a delicious ice cream sundae. Use ice cream made from pure ingredients, using the recipes in this book.

Our recipe for Hot Fudge Sundae Sauce is the basis for:

A VARIETY OF CAROB CONFECTIONS

Combine the cooled hot fudge sundae sauce with —

(1) Toasted sesame seeds;

(2) Chopped toasted Spanish peanuts (without skins);

(3) Chopped walnuts;

(4) Grated coconut;

(5) Ground or chopped almonds.

Make little balls or squares of this mixture and wrap in aluminum foil. Place in freezer where these candies will keep indefinitely. They make welcome gifts and are an ideal candy for children.

CAROB CANDY

2 cups honey
2 cups sunflower seeds, shelled
1/2 cup carob powder
1 1/2 cups almonds, shelled
2 cups sesame seeds, toasted
Rind of 1 large organic lemon*

Mix honey and carob powder thoroughly. Grind all other ingredients and add to honey mixture. Divide into teaspoon portions and wrap in wax paper or aluminum foil. Store in freezer.

*If you can't obtain an organic lemon, omit the rind.

This candy is non-fattening, nutritious, very rich in vitamins and minerals, and requires no cooking.

FROZEN "BANANA-SICLES"

Ripe bananas
Carob powder
Honey
Almond or sunflower seed meal
Popsicle sticks

Peel bananas, cut them into halves vertically and insert popsicle sticks into them. Roll the half bananas into syrup mixture made of carob powder and honey, then into almond meal or sunflower seed meal. Wrap each banana-sicle into waxed paper. Store in freezer for future use.

This makes a marvelous, nutritious, wholesome confection for the children as well as adults, instead of the harmful sugar candies. It is also an excellent way to use very ripe bananas.

BANANA-ALMOND-CAROB CONFECTION

Make the Hot Carob Fudge Sauce, the recipe for which you will find in this section. Then do the following:

Take a cupful of raw almonds and grind them rather coarsely in your seed and nut grinder, or chop them with a sharp knife on a bread board.

Spread the chopped almonds in a Pyrex pie plate. Slice two or three ripe bananas and put them over the ground almonds. Cover the two ingredients with the carob fudge sauce. Place in freezer. You will have a delicious frozen dessert, ready for all occasions. Eat with spoon.

Other varieties are possible, such as using chopped walnuts or grated coconut with the bananas and carob fudge sauce. Both children and adults should use these desserts instead of the commercial sweets made with chocolate, white sugar and artificial flavorings and chemicals.

ICE CREAM

Ice cream is a very popular dessert, but the ordinary, commercial ice cream is a terrible hodge-podge of sweetened chemical substances, with no resemblance to the good, old-fashioned home-made ice cream of yesteryear. (See Chapter XI — "You'd Be Surprised!")

Here are two ice cream recipes with only wholesome ingredients. From these, you can make your own adaptations, for other flavors.

STRAWBERRY ICE CREAM

1/2 cup almonds, ground and powdered
2 cups cream
3/4 cup honey
1/2 cup low-fat milk, soy or rice milk
1/2 cup toasted sesame seeds, ground and powdered
2 cups fresh strawberries or other fruit in season

Put milk, strawberries, honey, powdered nuts and seeds into your blender. Blend thoroughly and pour into refrigerator tray. Partially freeze to a mush consistency. Whip the cream in the blender and fold into the partially frozen mixture. Return to tray and freeze until firm.

HONEY-WALNUT ICE CREAM

1/2 cup scalded milk
2 cup yolks, beaten
1/2 cup cold milk
1 cup whipping cream
1/4 cup honey
1 cup chopped walnuts

Combine egg yolks with the 1/2 cup cold milk, honey and whipping cream. Slowly add this mixture to the now cooled scalded milk. Cook over hot water or in a double boiler until mixture coats spoon. Add walnuts. Cool slightly, then pour into ice cube tray (or similar-type pan) and let harden for 3 to 4 hours.

CRANBERRY SHERBET SUPREME

1 lb. cranberries
2 ripe bananas
Juice of 2 oranges
1 apple, peeled
3/4 cup honey, or to taste
1/2 cup cream (optional)

Pick over cranberries, rinse, and put into blender. Squeeze the two oranges and put juice into blender. Blend all ingredients until smooth. Turn into ice tray of refrigerator. Stir twice while freezing. Serve plain or garnish with slivered almonds or other ground nuts.

(If weight is not your problem, you may add 1/2 cup cream to the above ingredients.)

VARIATIONS: When cranberries are out of season, you could try other fruits — fresh or frozen — such as peaches, strawberries, oranges, etc.

With the same ingredients, and taking the steps through the blending, do not freeze. You can serve alone as a dessert, or can use as a topping over ice cream or pudding.

AVOCADO SHERBET

Pulp of 1 large avocado or 2 small avocados; rind of 1 organic lemon (or omit if not organic); 1/3 cup lemon juice; 1 cup milk; 4 TBS honey; 1/2 cup powdered almonds. Blend all ingredients until smooth. Turn into ice tray of refrigerator. Stir twice while freezing. Garnish with fruit to serve. Serves 6.

SMOOTHIE DELISH (Dairyless Ice Cream)

Peel, core and cut up any fruit in season. Freeze in a wooden or stainless steel bowl. Do the same with bananas in another bowl.

To make a quick, delicious, healthful dessert, simply mix 2 pints of frozen bananas and 1 pint assorted other frozen fruits, and run the mixture through a blender.

NUT MILK CUSTARD

3 eggs   1 tsp. honey
1 tsp. pure vanilla   2 cups almond nut milk
                                       (see recipe in this book)

Beat the eggs, then add the vanilla and the other ingredients. Beat all together. Pour into custard dishes (rubbed with sweet butter), and steam until the spoon comes out clear. Be careful not to cook too long.

PUMPKIN CUSTARD

2 cups fresh steamed pumpkin
    or 2 cups yellow winter squash
1/2 cup honey   4 eggs, slightly beaten
2 tsp. pumpkin pie spice   2 cups low-fat or soy milk

Mix pumpkin or squash with the honey and spices. Blend thoroughly and add the slightly beaten eggs and milk and mix well. Pour into eight buttered custard cups. Set cups in a baking pan with one or two inches of hot water. Bake at 300 degrees for 1 hour or until set.

SQUASH PUFF

3 cups cooked, mashed acorn squash
1/4 tsp. nutmeg
1/2 cup molasses
3 eggs, separated
3 TBS whole wheat flour
1/4 cup finely chopped pecans

In a large bowl, blend together squash, molasses, flour, nutmeg and egg yolks, Beat egg whites until stiff but not dry. Gently fold egg whites into squash mixture. Turn into a greased 1 1/2 quart round baking dish. Sprinkle pecans around outer edge. Bake at 350 degrees for one hour, or until top is golden brown and crusty. This dish is similar to pumpkin custard.

HONEY NUTS

Raw Spanish peanuts
Honey

Toast the peanuts under the broiler without burning them. The skins can be easily removed by rubbing the peanuts between the hands and by blowing and stirring them. Roughly chop the skinned nuts and then combine them with the honey. Eat with a spoon.

Variations: Chopped nuts, such as almonds, walnuts and filberts can be used instead of Spanish peanuts. Also, you may wish to combine toasted sesame seeds with honey.

This recipe is simple to make. A healthful, delicious confection, it is much better for children than those made of the harmful ingredients — sugar, chocolate, artificial colorings, and chemical preservatives.

SWEET-SOUR COMPOTE BOWL

(A delicious health breakfast or dessert)

Dried apricots, figs, prunes (any or all of these. Raisins, pure water, walnuts, almonds, or sunflower seeds, yogurt, soy or rice milk, low-fat milk, honey

Put hot bottled water over a bowlful of the above fruits. Let stand 48 hours out of the refrigerator, until all the fruit is soft.

To prepare the compote bowl, use the following:

FRESH FRUIT (peeled, cut into pieces) — pears and/or apples and/or bananas (no oranges.)

DRIED FRUIT COMPOTE on top of that.

Grind in your nut grinder any of these: walnuts, almonds, sunflower seeds.

Top with yogurt or milk (per above); add a little honey or pure maple syrup for sweetening if desired.

CANTALOUPE DE LUXE

1 ripe* cantaloupe
2/3 cup ground almonds
1/3 cup sesame seeds
Fresh lemon juice
2 tsp. honey
Raisins
1/2 cup unsweetened apple or pineapple juice

Cut the cantaloupe in half. Discard seeds and scoop out the hollow a little, to make more room for the nut and seed mixture. Blanch the almonds (see instructions under "Nuts" section). Toast the sesame seeds lightly, under broiler. Fine grind both the nuts and seeds together in your nut grinder, and put into small bowl. Add the honey and fruit juice; stir well. Squeeze a little lemon juice into mixture, to taste. If it seems too dry you may add more fruit juice. Scoop mixture into the hollows of the cantaloupe and garnish with a few raisins. Serves two.

This is a very filling dessert after a light meal. It may be served as the main dish (the *pièce de resistance*) for a Sunday or holiday breakfast.

*Make sure the cantaloupe is ripe. Much of the fruit purchased in the supermarket is not ripe; it does not taste good and lacks the nourishing qualities. If the cantaloupe is not ripe when you buy it leave it out of the refrigerator until it is very ripe. You can use an outdoor location or a drying cupboard.

Variation: Instead of the almonds and sesame seeds, you may use 1 cup sunflower seeds (hulled, raw, unsalted). Pick over and grind in nut grinder. Follow remainder of recipe. This is truly delicious, but does have a gray color, which may not be be so attractive, for a party.

CANTALOUPE A LA MODE

Fill the hollow of a ripe cantaloupe with our Strawberry Ice Cream.

DELICIOUS BANANA DESSERTS

HEALTH DRINK NO. 1 (BANANA-CARROT)

Fill your blender 2/3 full of carrot juice (home-made, preferably.) Add two bananas, sliced. Add 1/2 to 1 cup sunflower seeds (shelled, unsalted.) Blend. Pour into glasses.

HEALTH DRINK NO. 2 (BANANA-PEACH)

Put ripe, peeled peaches and ripe bananas into your blender and blend. Pour into glasses. This is smooth, delicious, very healthful — a rich, nourishing breakfast all by itself.

These drinks are also good for children after school, or for anyone hungry before bedtime. They are easy to digest.

INSTANT "HEALTHWAY" APPLESAUCE*

4 solid, ripe apples
1/2 tsp. cinnamon
1/2 cup pure apple juice
2 tsp. honey

Peel and cut the apples into small pieces. Put the apple juice into the blender, add half the apple chunks and blend to a thick consistency. Mix the remaining pieces of apple with the cinnamon and honey. Add this mixture to the liquefied apples and complete the blending. If any is left over, store in a glass jar in the refrigerator.

*Oxidation will turn this mixture dark but will not interfere with its nutritive value.

MAPLE SYRUP

You can use the pure, natural, wholesome maple syrup instead of the harmful white sugar in most places. It is excellent on bowls of cereal and/or fruit — a marvelously wholesome, nourishing dish, especially for children. Unfortunately, it is quite expensive.

The natural, pure Vermont maple syrup has no additives, no preservatives and no sugar added. Pure Vermont maple syrup is made from the sap of the state's native sugar maple tree.

Many of these trees are over 100 years old. Vermont maple syrup is produced only during the early spring by drilling a small hole in each tree from which gallons of sap drip each season. A combination of freezing nights and warm days is necessary. It takes from 40 to 50 gallons of sap, boiled down in an evaporator over a hot fire, to produce one gallon of pure Vermont maple syrup. This is why it is so expensive.

After opening the can or bottle, one should keep the maple syrup refrigerated. Freezing does not damage the product; it will retain its flavor longer.

MAPLE NUT FUDGE

2 cups pure maple syrup
1/2 cup light cream
1/2 cup chopped nuts

Mix the syrup and cream; cook until a few drops form a soft ball in cold water. Remove from heat, cool to 120 degrees, and stir until color changes. Add nuts, pour in buttered tin immediately.

MAPLE SYRUP FROSTING

1 cup pure maple syrup
2 eggs whites (beaten until stiff)

Cook maple syrup at 128 degrees. Pour in thin stream over the egg whites while beating continually. Spread when cool.

EYEBRIGHT DELIGHT

1 large bunch young carrots
1 cup ground sunflower seeds
1/2 cup apple juice or pineapple juice
1 cup raisins (organic preferred)
1/2 cup non-fat milk or soy milk or carrot juice

Scrape carrots and cut into small to medium-sized pieces. Put them into blender along with the liquids for easy blending. After blending, add the ground sunflower seeds, raisins and blend again. If desired, add more raisins on top, as a garnish.

HEALTH VALUES

This unusual, nourishing and delicious recipe is simplicity itself. It can be used as a main dish for a lunch, served on lettuce leaves for a salad (very nice topped with avocado), or as a dessert (topped with raisins).

Both carrots and sunflower seeds are known to aid eyesight. That is because they are rich in Vitamin A and B2, which are the vitamins that improve eyesight. This blended combination is soft, so it is marvelous for babies (use instead of canned vegetables) and for elderly who may have poor teeth. Versatile for your menus, you can make all kinds of variations.

CARROT CAKE DESSERT

Place two or three slices of Carrot Cake into a dish. Cover the cake with home-made ice cream. Then pour some low-fat milk over both.

This makes a very delicious dessert. The recipes for the carrot cake and the ice cream are in this chapter. Do not use any store-bought ice cream. Use only the ice cream you make yourself, from pure ingredients.

Variation: You may sprinkle some almond meal (ground almonds) over the entire mixture.

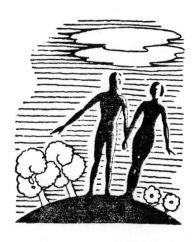

"Nothing in Nature, much less conscious being,
Was e'er created solely for itself."

—Edward Young

CHAPTER VIII

CORN, THE TRUE STAFF OF LIFE

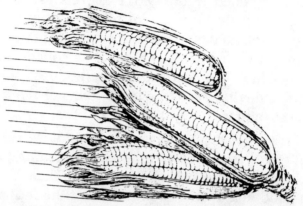

Among the foods included in the natural diet fresh corn-on-the cob is one of the best. This unique plant has not received the recognition it deserves as a component of the natural diet. In fresh form it is a vegetable; in dry form, it's a cereal.

Using this satisfying vegetable and cereal will help those who have difficulty in eliminating bread and other cooked starches from their diets. Wheat seems to be more generally popular, but in many tests corn has given better results. It gives more nourishment and is easier to digest.

Fresh corn has proved, in my life, to be such a valuable food that I have recommended it to a great number of people who have become equally enthusiastic about it. But note: when I refer to the high value of corn, I am not including canned, frozen, or processed corn.

It was deep in the midst of the past that Nature bestowed on Mankind the cereals which today provide the chief source of food for man and his domestic animals. Nature devised rice for the Oriental lands, the sorghum family for Africa and parts of Asia, and on the hills and plateaus of America she gave Man the best of all cereals — the botanically unique species that we call maize or Indian corn.

In the fifteenth century, when the wonders of the New World were opened to the Old, explorers found the native American cultivating this useful plant. Corn was the main food of the Indians who used it in its natural state to a much greater extent than it is used today. Of course, the Indians didn't "explode" it, flake it, make corn chips, or otherwise process it to death. Also, the other items of the Indian diet were used in a more natural state than ours.

Historic data tells of cases where Indians subsisted on corn and water, exclusively, for weeks or months, performing tasks which required great endurance. There is no doubt that the good health and good morals of the Indians (before they were corrupted by the white man's evil habits) resulted from their extensive use of the simple and natural foods, and their constant exposure to sunshine and fresh air.

Today, corn has the largest acreage of any grain in the New World. The principal reason that corn has such an extensive cultivation is its great value as stock feed, and the fact that it yields more grain per acre than any other cereal. The great development of the stock industry in the Middle West is due mainly to the abundant supply of corn for feed. Nine-tenths of the corn crop is fed directly to stock; the other one-tenth is manufactured into a great variety of products, the main ones being glucose, alcohol, and the so-called cereal foods. What little is used for human consumption is cooked, refined and processed so that nearly all its beneficial qualities are destroyed. (All except the sweet corn sold as fresh produce.)

In colonial days corn was an important article of food and was used extensively in both its natural and cooked state. However, with the development of wheat culture, commercialism and food distortion, corn has been almost entirely superseded by other grains for human consumption.

A chemical analysis of fresh corn shows that it contains considerable amounts of protein, carbohydrates, fats, natural sugar, water, mineral salts and vitamins. It is a good source of potassium, B vitamins, and fiber. This makes it one of the best balanced of the cereals and vegetables as a class.

It should be remembered that when corn is over-cooked, roasted or processed, the vitamins are destroyed, and the minerals and other food constituents are changed from an organic live form into an inorganic dead state. In that way these food elements are not only made useless as far as nourishing the human mechanism is concerned, but act as a clogging agent and a source of disease.

Properly prepared corn is surprisingly satisfying. It possesses a mild, delicious sweetness which is more highly appreciated the more one eats it. Corn combines nicely, and is compatible with, most of the other raw fruits and vegetables.

After making fresh corn an important staple of your diet, you will, when you are marketing, learn to distinguish the young ears from the old, the sweet from the tasteless, and the fresh from the left-overs. Try to find a source that has fresh corn from which the husks have not been removed. This is Nature's protective coat and it helps to maintain the corn's freshness.

Do not hesitate to give fresh corn to the children. Give them as much as they desire. It will develop their jawbones and teeth, as well as every other part of the body. Once they learn to appreciate the natural taste of this wonderful all-around food, properly prepared, they will reject the over-cooked, washed-out product, which has to be seasoned heavily with injurious condiments to make it palatable.

The correct preparation of fresh corn is of the utmost importance. It should be prepared with a minimum of cooking.

One can make a complete meal of the corn alone. It is important that only sweet, unsalted butter, and not ordinary salted butter, be used. Or use unsalted soy margarine. You may use a salt-free vegetable seasoning.

When suffering from arthritis, you must be careful about the water you drink and use in your diet. Use only bottled water, not tap or fluoridated water because of the harmful chemicals therein. Any foreign substance entering the body disturbs the delicate balance of metabolism and results in sickness and disease. Therefore, when dropping the fresh ears of corn into the water, use water as pure as possible, free from chemical pollutants.

In cases of diseased and inflamed conditions of the mouth due to hyperacidity, a diet made up predominantly of fresh corn, for a short while, is very curative.

In cases of arthritis, the use of fresh corn is of great value. Even in cases of ulcers of the stomach, where roughage is not well tolerated, fresh corn has proven very compatible.

Considering its physical properties, its laxative effect, its chemical and physiological effects, fresh corn ranks as one of the leaders of the natural foods. Actually, the corn kernels are seeds. Could this be the corn's source of power, in being such a marvelous food for man?

With me it holds a place that no other plant can fill. I eat it every day of the entire season, and when it leaves the market I feel as though a good friend and humble servant has departed for a year's journey.

PREPARATION OF SWEET CORN

SWEET CORN ON THE COB

One of the finest foods you can eat is corn on the cob, if properly prepared. It should not be cooked "to death."

Choose fresh *young* ears. Try to buy them in husks, and leave in husks until ready to prepare.

Nature has supplied this vegetable with a little protecting coat—against insects, the elements—too much sunshine, rain, cold—and against drying out.

Boil enough water to cover the ears, using a large pot with a well fitting cover. Turn off the heat.

Remove the husks and place the corn into the hot water, without cooking it. Let the corn soak in the hot water for about five minutes, before serving.

To season the corn, rub a little unsalted butter over the hot ears, or you may use a seasoning made with a mixture of Brewers' yeast, kelp and garlic powder. The proportions, which may be varied, are: 1/2 cup Brewers' yeast powder; 1 teaspoon kelp powder; 1 teaspoon garlic powder.

It is best to make a complete meal of the corn, alone.

In warm weather, if the corn is young and sweet, it can be eaten raw, without any heating. Keep out of the refrigerator before eating.

Corn comes in two main varieties, and there is a marked difference between them. Sweet corn is for human consumption, and field corn is for animal consumption. Field corn is coarser and tougher, with large kernels. Yes, it is sold in supermarkets, so watch out for it. Choose the young ears with small kernels.

Also, remember the use of corn meal, which is versatile and wholesome. You can make corn bread, corn sticks, corn meal mush, and polenta (another word for the mush). The polenta can be further developed into fancier dishes. Consult your cookbooks for more corn and corn meal recipes, but delete the ingredients you now know are harmful.

POPPED CORN

The popcorn sold in movie houses should be avoided. Both the salt and the heated oil used are harmful to everyone, but especially to arthritis sufferers.

If you must have popcorn, prepare it at home in an *air* popper. Add no salt or butter. Microwave popcorn is to be avoided; much of it has up to 50 percent fat.

CHAPTER IX

THE APPLE — QUEEN OF FRUITS

(Nature's Blessing for Arthritis Sufferers)

We consider the apple one of the most important fruits — for three reasons: (1) It is a delicious food that agrees with people of all ages; (2) It is highly nutritious, packed with essential organic minerals and vitamins, and has a therapeutic effect on arthritis; (3) It is available all year round

FIRST: Apples grow abundantly and in many varieties, with many flavors to suit all tastes. They make an enjoyable, healthful snack. They combine with other fruits to make a delicious fruit bowl. (See recipe section.)

SECOND: Apples contain a high percentage of Vitamin C for the health of the skin, teeth, gums, bones and joints. Vitamin C also helps in the healing of wounds and the prevention of colds. Apples are very beneficial in cases of arthritis.

Apples are a rich source of important organic minerals — especially calcium, phosphorus and magnesium.

The calcium is important for building and maintaining healthy bones and teeth. It helps the blood to clot and thus prevents excessive bleeding. Calcium also aids the body with vitality and endurance and regulates the rhythm of the heart. The phosphorus is interrelated with the calcium, and both work together to perform the above functions. The magnesium serves to enhance the calcium and Vitamin C metabolism. It is essential for the normal function of the nervous and muscular system. Magnesium is the key mineral that prevents the formation of stones in the urinary system.

Thus we can see why apples so truly deserve the famous old saying, "An apple a day keeps the doctor away." We eat apples every day.

The apple is also called "Nature's toothbrush," because it has a cleansing effect on the teeth and the entire intestinal tract.

After eating lunch at school, children often finish it with a sugary, sweet dessert — candy, etc. This, of course, causes dental caries (cavities). Very few children brush their teeth after lunch at school. So, give school children an apple in their lunch bags, teaching them to end their lunches with the cleansing apple.

In choosing apples, you should remember that there is a vast difference in quality. Those picked before well ripened and then treated with chemical sprays and finally waxed, are not good to eat. The apples you should eat are those that have been tree-ripened and not treated or embalmed with chemicals to prevent spoilage. Try to get organically-grown apples from health food stores, or from a small organic orchard.

THIRD: Finally, the other reason why apples are so important a food is that they are available all year around.

During the winter months, when most of the other fruits are out of season, apples are available and that is a godsend.

APPLES FOR ALL AGES

Besides being an excellent food for arthritics, apples are good for all ages. Children will thrive better if you give them an apple instead of a cookie or candy bar for a snack. Hopefully, they will retain the habit when older. The majority of American teen-agers have atrocious, injurious eating habits, and these were formed in childhood.

For Babies: Liquefied apples are wonderful to balance the baby's diet. They prevent eating too many starchy foods and also furnish the essential minerals and vitamins. If you do not have a blender, just cut the apple in half, and scoop and scrape the apple with a spoon. Babies love it, especially the sweet red Delicious apple.

Another good reason for using apples and other fruits for babies is to give them a wholesome, natural food, in place of the canned baby foods, many of which are loaded with sugar, salt and preservatives.

As written in Chapter IV, arthritis formerly was considered a disease of mature and elderly people, but now young children are being crippled with it. The reason for this is the increased use of canned foods for babies. If you want your child to avoid arthritis, feed him fresh, natural foods, instead of canned or bottled foods, and "junk foods."

Most vegetables can be steamed and mashed for babies and young children. Mashed ripe bananas are excellent.

Fresh, natural food is not only more healthful — it is more economical than canned foods.

SUGGESTIONS FOR CHOOSING APPLES

In choosing your apples, quality is of great importance. *Quality* does *not* depend upon *price*. There are various ways to judge the quality of an apple:

1. COLOR: The deeper the color, the more nourishing and better-tasting the apple will be. If you want to convince yourself, take two apples, one light-colored with areas of green and only a small amount of red color. Then take another, with a *full red color*. Taste both, and you will realize how much better the deep-colored apple is. Not only is the taste better, but more important, the nourishment is superior. The test of color is true even for the green Pippin. The more yellow the color, the sweeter the Pippin.

There are many varieties of apples. Our first choice is the Red Delicious. When these are not available, our next choice is the McIntosh, and then the Baldwin.

2. FEEL: This is another way to judge a fruit. If the apple is hard and does not "give" when pressed with the finger, then it means one of two things — either the fruit was picked too soon before it was ripe, or it was embalmed with

a biphenol chemical so that it will never spoil. Such apples are not good to eat.

Another feature to look for is the waxing of fruit. Often you can feel the waxy surface, especially if you pour some hot water over the fruit. The hot water will melt the wax, but will not remove it. The only way to avoid eating the wax is to peel the fruit.

3. ODOR: If you have a good sense of smell, you may be able to detect the chemicals with which the fruit has been treated. By letting the hot water run on the calyx of the apple, the odor is accentuated. (The calyx is the end opposite the stem.)

4. TASTE: The final test for quality of a fruit is the taste. A good food tastes good, not only while you are eating it, but also should not leave a bad taste *after* eating.

NOTE: Just because an apple looks red, large, and perfect, does not mean that it is wholesome. As a rule, the organic apples look rustic and imperfect. You must consider as well the hardness, the taste, and the odor.

Our editor had this experience on a flight to Europe: Being a person devoted to these principles of natural health who doesn't eat sugar, she requested fruit instead of the usual sugary dessert. A large, red, perfect-looking Delicious apple was served to her. She did not eat it, but kept it during her stay in Scotland. One month later, it looked just the same — as perfect, but hard as a rock. It had not spoiled, because it was embalmed. She did not eat it. Watch out for the embalming and waxing of apples. You will be taking into your body chemicals that do not belong there!

All of this food-testing may seem complicated to you now, but after a while you will become an expert at judging foods. You will do this automatically, with very little effort. It will pay big dividends in good health.

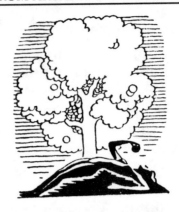

The boy is indeed the true apple-eater, and is not to be questioned how he came by the fruit with which his pockets are filled. It belongs to him. . . . His own juicy flesh craves the juicy flesh of the apple. Sap draws sap. His fruit-eating has little reference to the state of his appetite. Whether he be full of meat or empty of meat he wants the apple just the same. Before meal or after meal it never comes amiss. The farm boy munches apples all day long. He has nests of them in the hay-mow, mellowing, to which he makes frequent visits. Sometimes old Brindle, having access through the open door, smells them out and makes short work of them.

In some countries the custom remains of placing a rosy apple in the hand of the dead that they may find it when they enter paradise. In northern mythology the giants eat apples to ward off old age.

The apple is indeed the fruit of youth. As we grow old we crave apples less. It is an ominous sign. When you are ashamed to be seen eating them on the street; when you can carry them in your pocket and your hand does not constantly find its way to them; when your neighbor has apples and you have none, and you make no nocturnal visits to his orchard; when your lunch-basket is without them, and you can pass a winter's night by fireside with no thought of the fruit at your elbow, then be assured that you are no longer a boy, either in heart or years.

CHAPTER X

PART I

THE New Four Food Groups

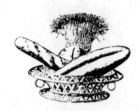

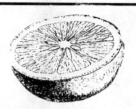

Generations of wide-eyed school-children have dutifully memorized the USDA'S dietary guidelines, popularized in the 1950's as the "Four Food Groups." These "Basic Four" have been the major source of nutrition education for 35 years. They have found their way into almost every Home Ec classroom in the country and are probably as much a part of Americana as baseball and apple pie.

But the Basic Four will be on their way out the door if the Physicians Committee for Responsible Medicine has its way. On April 8, 1991, PCRM made a proposal to the U. S. Department of Agriculture (USDA) to change its food groupings from meat, fruits/vegetables, dairy products, and bread and cereal to four new healthful groups: whole grains, vegetables, legumes, and fruits. Meat and dairy products lose their food group status and become options under the new plan.

PCRM was joined by notable experts Denis Burkitt, M.D., the world renowned physician who discovered the value of fiber in the diet; T. Colin Campbell, Ph. D. of Cornell University, who heads the ground-breaking China Health project; and Oliver Alabaster, M.D., a cancer researcher at George Washington University.

"Over the years, the Four Food Groups took on the air of a sanctioned requirement. But it tends to sustain something we ought not be doing— eating a diet high in animal fat and protein and lacking in fiber," said Dr. Campbell. His ongoing study of diet and nutrition in China has demonstrated the dramatic effects of a plant-based diet in cutting the risk factors for heart disease, cancer and stroke, the major killers of Americans.

"I support the idea of shifting emphasis away from the present four food groups," said Dr. Alabaster. "Meat and dairy products are high in fat, which is associated with increased risk of cancer and heart disease. We have the ability to save both lives and money by making major changes in our diet, and this is one way to do it."

163

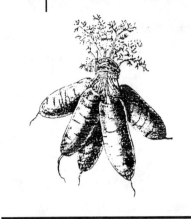
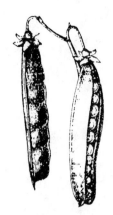

Dr. Burkitt, who has done extensive research in Africa, said that although developed countries have steadily increased intake of meat and dairy products over the last 200 years, our bodies really have no more use for these foods than they did 20,000 years ago.

"Everybody in America has a Stone Age body," Burkitt said. "What we are doing is putting high grade fuel into engines made to run on diesel."

Shortly after PCRM's conference, the USDA announced that it was changing the format for the presentation of the food groups from its old "food wheel" to the "Eating Right Pyramid." The wheel gave equal emphasis to all of the food groups, while the pyramid design de-emphasizes meat and dairy products considerably.

Nutritionists applauded; livestock producers fumed. And a few days later the USDA caved in to the meat and dairy producers and pulled back the pyramid—after three years of research and dialogue with consumers.

This has provoked much criticism from many different groups, including the American Cancer Society, the Society for Nutrition Education, and the Center for Science in the public Interest. All have written to the USDA requesting that it reconsider the decision.

The irony is that the food pyramid was a very modest change. PCRM's New Four Food Groups is a much more potent alternative to the Basic Four. Numerous scientific studies over the last 35 years have yielded more than enough evidence to recommend a dramatic shift in America's eating habits.

A poster of the New Four Food Groups is available from PCRM for $5.00. Send a check or money order to PCRM,
P.O. Box 6322,
Washington, D.C. 20015.

By Melissa Goldman
from "A Guide to Healthy Eating,"
Physicians Committee for
Responsible Medicine.
PO Box 6322
Washington, D. C. 20015

PART II

FACTS ON VITAMINS

VITAMIN A — Found in: Butter, Raw Milk, Egg Yolk, Yellow Vegetables such as Pumpkin, Yellow Squash, Sweet Potatoes, Yams, Carrots, and Yellow fruits.

Good for: Eyes, Skin, Hair, Organs and Glands.

VITAMIN B — Found in: Rice, Bran, Wheat Germ, Whole Wheat, Oatmeal, Nuts, Peanuts, Raw Milk, Yeast, Vegetables.

Good for: Growth, Digestion and Nerves.

VITAMIN C — Found in: Citrus Fruits, Green Vegetables, Raw Tomatoes, Cabbage, Spinach, Lettuce and Potatoes.

Good for: Skin, Teeth, Gums, Bones, Joints. Promotes wound healing. Helps prevent capillary fragility.

VITAMIN D — Found in: Sunshine; Green leafy vegetables, grown in the sunshine.

Good for: Teeth, Bones, Nerves, Calcium, Phosphorus and Iron Metabolism.

VITAMIN E — Found in: Egg Yolk, Whole Grain Cereals, Wheat Germ, Wheat Germ Oil, Lettuce, Corn on the Cob, Sesame Seeds, Soya Beans.

Good for: Heart, General Well-being, Vitality and Energy.

IMPORTANT MINERALS

CALCIUM — Found in: Raw Milk, Cheese, Sunflower Seeds, Raw Almonds, Raw Cabbage.

Good for: Building and maintaining bones and teeth; Helping blood to clot; Aiding vitality and endurance; Regulating heart rhythm.

PHOSPHORUS — Found in: Whole Grains, Sunflower Seeds, Raw Nuts, Sea Foods, Vegetables and Potatoes.

Good for: Normal bone and tooth structure. Inter-related with action of Calcium and Vitamin D.

IRON — Found in: Spinach, Apricots, Kale, Molasses, Raisins, Nuts and Parsley.

Good for: Production of hemoglobin; Helping to carry oxygen to the blood.

IODINE — Found in: Kelp, Onions, Artichokes and Sea Foods.

Good for: The proper function of the thyroid gland; Essential for proper growth, energy and metabolism.

MAGNESIUM Found in: Sesame, Sunflower and Pumpkin Seeds, Nuts, Peanuts, Soy Beans, Barley, Asparagus, Corn, Lettuce, Lima Beans, Peas, String Beans and Apples.

Good for: Calcium and Vitamin C metabolism; essential for normal functioning of nervous and muscular system. It is the key mineral that prevents the formation of stones in the body.

VEGETABLE PROTEINS

Vegetable Proteins are found in:

All the Nuts (Almonds, first choice; Walnuts and Pecans are good; Cashews are not recommended. All nuts should be fresh and raw, not roasted or salted.)

All the Seeds (the best being Sunflower, Sesame and Pumpkin.)

All the Beans (Soy; String; Lima; Navy; Garbanzo, etc.) Sprouts; Millet and Whole Grain Cereals; Lentils; Peas; Peanuts.

Avocados

BASIC NATURAL FOODS

In any area where the supply of fruit and vegetables is scarce, one can get along nicely with a *few* good, natural foods, such as apples, potatoes, onions, carrots, cabbage and *sprouts*. The sprouts take the place of fresh vegetables, and furnish us with a remarkable storehouse of health-giving vitamins, minerals, and complete proteins. Be sure to read the chapter on SPROUTS. There you will learn how to regain and maintain your health with only a *few natural foods*, at a *very low cost*. There you will find the *key* to combatting arthritis, no matter where you live, and no matter how poor you are.

The Unique Potassium Herbal Formula

> "For a lifetime it has helped me, my family, and friends. In 60 years, I have never seen this product fail once in doing some good for the people using it."
>
> —*Dr. Karl Jurak, Creator of Km.*

 is an herbal formula developed in 1922 in Austria by Dr. Karl Jurak to give him more strength and endurance for his studies and for his favorite sport, mountain climbing. He was awarded a Doctorate degree with honors at the age of 19, in agrobiology (the study of plant biology) for the discovery of his elixir, which we now know as Km.

Interestingly, the key to the catalyst, which eluded him during his 9 months of study, appeared to him in a dream, and completed his formula.

His preparation contains chamomile flowers, sarsaparilla root, celery seed, angelica root, dandelion root, horehound root, licorice, senega root, passion flower, thyme, gentian root, saw palmetto berry, alfalfa and cascara sagrada. All these plants have special healthful properties, some of them used for many ages in different parts of the world, and by Indians. But he did not merely combine them—it was a special *synergy* that made the unique formula. Due to his extensive knowledge of plants, Dr. Jurak was able to actually work with the molecular structure of plants. He said, "If you change even one molecule of the plant, the whole effect is changed." It is a formula that cannot be duplicated. Each of these plants is rich in vital nutrients: vitamins, minerals and essential trace minerals.

Dr. Jurak gave his elixir away to friends and family for forty years and then passed the formula on to his son, who then continued to help others with its benefits. Up until a few years ago, you would have had to be a personal friend of the Juraks to obtain this "liquid health." Now, due to the system of network marketing (in the U.S. and Canada only), you can experience the benefits of Km today.

The Km herbal preparation can help you with your personal health. The unique formula of Km, as part of a healthful diet, can help you, like thousands of others, to have *the abundant energy and health you need.*

TO ORDER, CALL 800-350 LIFE

 is a blend of 14 special, beautiful herbs, in a potassium mineral liquid base. MANY PERSONS TODAY IN THE U.S. AND CANADA ARE ENJOYING Km.

Wachters!

Products from "The Garden of the Sea"

Neptune's Medicine Chest—The origin and success of **Wachters' Organic Sea Products**

The story behind Wachters' Organic Sea Products is a very interesting and unusual one. Just after the turn of the century, Joseph V. Wachter, a promising young pianist, learned that his severe lung condition was probably terminal. Determined to enjoy his last days to the fullest, Wachter journeyed to the most rugged and remote areas of the world. In Alaska, with his health at its lowest point, fate took a dramatic turn.

The local Indian people nursed him back to health. Their treatment consisted of using seaweeds primarily. They made a seaweed gruel for him to eat; they burned seaweed in a sweat lodge, for him to breathe in the healthful, natural ingredients. They also applied seaweed to his body. Wachter got well! After his cure, he devoted the rest of his life to studying marine vegetation. In 1932, Wachter and his wife Margaret began their company, which is now one of the largest in researching, refining, and distributing products from the sea. They had two sons who have carried on the business. Both are health professionals. The Wachter line has grown to over 100 products. It now includes food supplements for energy and blood building, intestinal cleansing, and cell supplementation; teas of herbal and sea vegetable combinations; soaps, shampoos, and skin creams; household cleansing products, and plant and agricultural products. These products are sold only through individual local distributors.

Internal Cleansing is the first step for the establishment and maintenance of positive good health.

—Dr. Joseph V. Wachter, Jr. (D. C.)

TO CLEANSE THE COLON: *Sea-Klenz Powder* (51-B) and *Intesti-Klenz Tablets* (96-A). Non-habit forming, vegetable, eliminates toxins, provides bulk factors, will not overstimulate like a purgative oral laxative but gently sweeps and conditions your digestive tract; encapsulates and removes mucoid wastes. Ingredients are: Sodium Alginate (from sea vegetation); Plantago Ovata Blond; Dehydrated Lemon Powder, Apple and Prune Powder; Wachters' Blend of Marine Algae.

FOR REFRESHING ENERGY: *Wachters' Sea Green Drink.* A unique combination of Vitamin C, Alfalfa Juice Concentrate, the Wachters' Blend of Sea Plants, Chlorophyll, Aloe Vera, Chlorella, Lemon Bioflavinoids, Rose Hips, Hesperidin Complex, Acerola, Rutin, and a good quantity of Carotene. A powder concentrate. Here is a real pepper-upper for energy during the day. *Sea Green Drink* is delicious, and possesses all those magic qualities of fresh, vibrant life.

All Wachters' Organic Sea Products are the result of this life process that benefits man: *FROM SUN TO SEA TO CELL.*

WHOLESOME, SALT-FREE SEASONING: Dr. Philip J. Welsh proved that the use of salt is one of the prime causes of arthritis. Now you can use a delicious, salt-free seasoning at home—Wachters No. 7 *Sea and Land Vegetable Seasoning.* Ingredients: Wachters' blend of sea plants, garlic, carrots, onions, tomatoes, peas, celery green peppers, green beans, parsley.

ENJOY TEA WITHOUT HARMFUL CAFFEINE AND TANNIN. USE WACHTERS' HERBAL-ALGAE TEAS—Yan Tsai Mint Sea Tea, and Almond Mist Sea Tea.

To order, call 800-350-LIFE

CHAPTER XI

YOU'D BE SURPRISED
AT WHAT YOU MAY BE EATING TODAY!

The following menu is translated into the *preservatives and additives* likely to be contained in the very foods you may be eating today.

Here is what you could be eating for LUNCH or DINNER:

JUICE:

Benzoic Acid	preservative
Dimethyl polysiloxane	anti-foaming agent

FRUIT CUP:

Calcium hypochlorite	germicide wash
Sodium chloride	prevents browning
Sodium hydroxide	peeling agent
Calcium hydroxide	firming agent
Sodium metasilicate	peeling agent for peaches
Sorbic acid	fungistat
Sulfur dioxide	preservative
FD&C Red No. 3	coloring for cherries

SOUP:

Butylated hydroxyanisole	anti-oxidant
Dimethyl polysiloxane	anti-foaming agent
Sodium phosphate dibasic	emulsion for tomato soup
Citric acid	dispersant in soup base

SANDWICH WITH MEAT AND PROCESSED CHEESE:

Sodium diacetate	mold inhibitor
Mono-glyceride	emulsifier
Potassium bromate	maturing agent
Aluminum phosphate	improver
Calcium phosphate monobasic	dough conditioner
Aluminum potassium sulfate	acid-baking powder ingredient

Ascorbate	anti-oxidant
Sodium or potassium nitrate	color fixative
Sodium chloride	preservative
Guar gum	binder
Hydrogen peroxide	bleach and bactericide
FD&C Yellow No. 3	coloring
Nordihydroguaiaretic acid	anti-oxidant
Alkanate	dye
Methylviolet	marking ink
Asafoetide	onion flavoring
Sodium phosphate	buffer
Magnesium carbonate	drying agent
Calcium propionate	preservative
Calcium citrate	plasticiser
Sodium citrate	emulsifier
Sodium alginate	stabilizer
Acetic acid	acid
Phroligneous acid	smoke flavor
Chloramine T	flour bleach
Chloramine T	deodorant

FRUIT PIE:

Sodium diacetate	mold inhibitor
Sorbic Acid	fungistat
Butylated hydroxyanisole	anti-oxidant
Sodium sulfite	anti-browning
Mono-and-di-glycerides	emulsifier
Aluminum ammonium sulfate	acid
FD&C Red No. 3	cherry coloring
Calcium Chloride	apple pie mix firming agent
Potassium bromate	maturing agent
Calcium carbonate	neutralizer

COMMERCIAL ICE CREAM:

(a) Dietheyl Glycol: Used instead of eggs, it is an anti-freeze and paint remover;

(b) Piperonal: Used in place of vanilla, it is a lice killer;

(c) Ethyl Acetate: Used in place of pineapple, it is a cleaner for leather and textiles;

(d) Butyraldehyde: Used instead of nuts, it is one of the ingredients of rubber cement;

(e) Amyl Acetate: Used for banana flavor; an oil paint solvent;

(f) Benzyl Acetate: Used for strawberry flavor; a solvent.

Do you know that you can make a delicious and healthful ice-milk by using any of the following ingredients: Milk, honey, fresh fruit, pure vanilla, and carob powder for chocolate flavoring?

After reading about the many chemical additives that are put into our foods, you can see why so many people are suffering with arthritis — as well as cancer and many other diseases. Over 3,000 additives are used in the manufacture of the food we eat. Some estimates of individual consumption are as high as five pounds per year! The Department of Consumer Affairs receives many letters and calls from consumers who are concerned about these additives. Even experts cannot agree on the safety of or necessity for all these chemicals.

AN INFORMATIVE PERIODICAL

We recommend that you subscribe to the *Natural Food and Farming* journal, published by Natural Food Associates. This newspaper will give you a wealth of highly important information contributed by some of the nation's foremost nutritionists.

The subscription price for the bi-monthly journal is $20.00 for one year. The address is: N.F.A., P. O. Box 210, Atlanta, TX 75551

In addition to a variety of informative articles each month, there are natural food recipes, book reviews, and a list of sources for obtaining unprocessed foods.

The July 1980 edition contained an important, revealing article entitled "The Poisons in Your Food," which tells about the hormone Diethylstilbestrol which, although it has been banned by the government, is still being used by thousands of cattlemen to fatten the cattle before slaughter. It has been proved to be carcinogenic (cancer-causing).

Another article tells about the dangers of using cortisone in the treatment of arthritis. It describes the terrible side effects resulting from the use of this drug, such as: depression of the adrenal glands, Addison's Disease, peptic ulcers, loss of judgement and severe eye damage.

We have received reports from readers who have suffered severe damages from cortisone treatments.

Nora Joyce, widow of the famous Irish writer, James Joyce, suffered with arthritis, was treated with cortisone, and died.

Recently, we saw an old movie, called "Bigger Than Life." Based on a true story, it told of the period when cortisone first was used. Cortisone was prescribed for a man with a serious illness, but it caused him to become psychotic; he almost killed his young son. He is rescued in time from the drug, and the film has a happy ending.

CHAPTER XII

OTHER AUTHORITIES AGREE
"FOOD IS YOUR BEST MEDICINE"

Fortunately, a *few* medical doctors are working along the same lines that I have recommended for fifty years — a change of diet — which brings almost miraculous results.

Henry G. Bieler, M.D., was one of these. In his book, *Food is Your Best Medicine*, he urged proper food instead of drugs to prevent and cure disease. The following is a quotation from this book:

"As a practicing physician for over fifty years, I have reached three basic conclusions as to the cause and cure of disease. This book is about those conclusions.

"The first is that the primary cause of disease is toxemia.

"My second conclusion is that in almost all cases the use of drugs in treating the patient is harmful. Drugs often cause serious side effects, and sometimes even create new diseases. The dubious benefits they afford the patient are at best temporary. Yet the number of drugs on the market increases geometrically every year as each chemical firm develops its own variation of the compounds . . . .

"My third conclusion is that disease can be cured through the proper use of correct foods . . . .

"My conclusions are based on experimental and observational results, gathered through years of successfully treating patients . . . .

"This book deals with what I consider to be the best food and the best medicine."

In his introduction, Dr. Bieler writes:

" . . . Today we are not only in the Atomic Age but also the Antibiotic Age (anti-biotic means "anti-life"!—Editor). Unhappily, too, this is the Dark Age of Medicine — an age in which many of my colleagues, when confronted with a patient, consult a volume which rivals the Manhattan telephone directory in size. This book contains the names of thousands upon thousands of drugs used to alleviate the distressing symptoms of a host of diseased states of the body. The doctor then decides which pink or purple or baby-blue pill to prescribe for the patient.

"This is not, in my opinion, the practice of medicine.

"Far too many of these new 'miracle' drugs are introduced with fanfare and then revealed as lethal (*deadly*) in character, to be silently discarded for newer and more powerful drugs, which allegedly cure all the ills to which the flesh is heir.

"I discarded drugs partly because I began to re-examine an old medical truism — that nature does the real healing, utilizing the natural defenses of the body. Under the proper conditions, nature, if given the opportunity, is always the greatest healer. It is the physician's role to assist in this healing — to co-operate with nature's forces; to play a supporting role instead of wanting to be star of the show. Nature does not follow Madison Avenue's 'Feel Better Faster' slogan, but takes her time, slowly, as a tree grows, a little more each day. Nature never rushes to get a sick man or beast on his feet; she demands a slow and steady convalescence. Sick animals rest or sleep and refuse all food until nature has healed them.

"Isn't it proper, then, to expect that nature can do the same thing for a sick human if only she is given the opportunity? . . . Briefly stated, my position is: improper foods cause disease; proper foods cure disease . . . . "

"A NEW BREED OF DOCTOR"

Alan H. Nittler, M.D., wrote a book entitled *A New Breed of Doctor.* Here is another medical authority whose ideas coincide with ours, and who is getting better results in curing many illnesses via nutrition.

Linda Clark, M.A., nutrition reporter, wrote the Foreword. We quote: "The average doctor is not taught this new science, which we call nutrition." (Actually, the Nature Cure pioneers, many of them M.D.'s, started this "new science" over 100 years ago, but most of the medical profession paid no attention to this new development.)

"Instead, the average doctor uses drugs which serve as a crutch or to mask the symptoms of disease. The science of nutrition, on the other hand, actually rebuilds the body . . . Alan H. Nittler, M.D., helps his patients rebuild their bodies. He does not use a drug except in dire emergencies. I have personally witnessed five lives that he has saved, some of them in an amazingly short time. I have also seen energy and good health return to patients even after years of suffering. . . ."

Dr. Nittler states in his courageous book: "I have come to know and believe absolutely that degenerative conditions of the body are usually nutritional in origin." He turned from drugs to nutrition.

He wrote: "I found that my patients were getting better, and I was getting more lasting and safer results than with the drugs I had previously used . . . . I continue to learn more about this new-found and growing science: *nutritional therapy.*"

"TOXEMIA EXPLAINED"

A pioneering authority who demonstrated the efficacy of a proper diet in the cure of disease was J. H. Tilden, M.D. He was one of the first medical doctors to take up natural methods of healing, and was highly successful in effecting cures in his sanatorium, and through his many fine writings. One of his major books, *"Toxemia Explained,"* is still available.

In his book, *"Impaired Health,"* Dr. Tilden wrote:

"It should be remembered that while people continue to eat, their digestive tracts and eliminative organs get no rest. To rest the entire body and give *Nature* a chance to heal, we should do as the animals do when sick or injured, and abstain from all food until well. Thus, the energy that is ordinarily utilized in digesting and assimilating three meals a day is available for cleansing the system of toxins, which in most of us have been gradually accumulating through years of wrong living. Fasting prepares the body for the health-gaining, rebuilding process which will follow if a more natural, healthful program of living is adopted. Above all, remember that the more you feed a diseased body, the more you feed the disease. So, first cleanse the body."

"DIETETIC ERRORS — A CAUSE OF ARTHRITIS"

George S. Weger, M.D., one of Dr. Tilden's disciples, wrote: "What, then, really is the cause of rheumatic arthritis? Our conviction is that the cause is primarily and fundamentally toxemia, which is brought about by dietetic errors and the accumulating effect of many little dissipations that are ordinarily considered harmless or of minor consequence . . . .

"Excessive coffee drinking in adults predisposed to rheumatism invites disaster when near the fortieth year. There is chemical proof to the effect that caffeine is converted into uric acid in the body . . . . Uric acid, instead of being the sole cause of rheumatism, is only one of the many acids (an excess of) which leads to trouble . . . ."

(Note: A high protein flesh diet causes excessive uric acid in the body.)

From "ARTHRITIS" by Victor P. Fleming, M.D.

After stating that 'toxemia' is the real cause of arthritis (as Drs. Tilden, Weger, and Bieler have done), Dr. Fleming wrote as follows:

DIETARY FACTOR

"Arthritis is essentially a condition of perverted or changed body chemistry. Over-indulgence in starches and sugars is the outstanding dietetic error and most active factor in altering the body chemistry to prepare it for arthritis. . . .

"The *real cause* of arthritis is *toxemia* brought about by *faulty diet and enervating habits of living,* and it is correction of these that makes the relief or cure of the condition possible in almost every case."

Now it should be easier for you to understand why the simple plan in this manual is so effective in conquering arthritis. Briefly, it entails the following:

(1) A brief fast; (2) The cleansing process; (3) The mono diet; (4) The addition of one food at a time. This is a very effective way of screening your foods to find out which foods aggravate the arthritis.

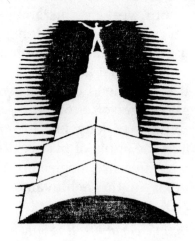

"The natural alone is permanent."

—Henry Wadsworth Longfellow

CHAPTER XIII

A LIFE FREE FROM SUFFERING

*"The dinner hour is a sacred part of the day . . . for it is
then that you are building the human temple."* — P.J.W.

We are all searching for a Life Supreme . . . a splendid, unhampered, constructive life . . . free from discordant, unhappy, unnatural conditions. Such a life is a priceless gift worthy of the greatest effort to achieve it. So, the question arises: What is this keystone of success and happiness, this greatest of all assets, this source of power, vigor, energy, and originality? What is this best friend to man? What is this blessing that is sought by both rich and poor? What is this great multiplier of ability . . . this backbone of self-confidence and enthusiasm?

It is the greatest constructive power in the life of man, without which his faith weakens, his ambition diminishes, his courage faints, his self-confidence departs, his accomplishments are nil. Without it, ambition and wealth are but a mockery . . . a palatial home and luxuries an empty disappointment. It is the friend of progress, the stimulator of ambition, the encourager of effort, the greatest essential for success, the promoter of long life and happiness. The wise man guards it as the apple of his eye; the fool abuses it through ignorance, indifference, neglect, or weakness. What is this greatest factor in the achievement of all that is worthwhile? It is GOOD HEALTH.

*"Without Health, Life is not life; it is only a state of
languor and suffering — an image of death."* — Rabelais

Daily we read in the newspapers of men successful in the world, who die at an early age. They have worked, conquered and at last arrived, only to stay but a short while on this earth. Is it not a pity that brilliant, learned men, outstanding leaders in their particular fields of endeavor,

180

masters of their chosen work, have not as yet mastered the art of arts, the science of all sciences, the one great business of all businesses — that of living, intelligent living, healthful living, natural living? Nothing is intelligent and healthful unless it is natural.

The scientist Pasteur examined all his food through a microscope, and then cooked and sterilized it before he consumed it. He concentrated on the laws of *Man* and overlooked the laws of *Nature*. He did not *know himself*, for he was an invalid the greater part of his life. He never knew the joys of the art of *natural living* . . . of good health.

Does it pay to work, plod, plan, build, and finally arrive, only to find that we must leave our hard-earned achievement but a short time after we have arrived? Is it efficiency to gain at one end and lose at the other? Is it wise to build all our days, merely to find, after the structure is complete, that we cannot live in it because our health and life have deserted us?

Few people realize how important the art of eating is; few give serious thought to their mode of feeding their bodies; few even know how closely health, efficiency, and the enthusiasm to carry on are related to one's mode of eating. Few realize that *a person is what he eats* — that he can eat his way to health — or that he can eat his way to death!

The human structure consists of a vast number of cells. There are only two sources from which the material for these cells can be obtained, and no others. They are AIR and FOOD. Cut off either of these two sources of supply and death results. Even interfere with them and disease and death are the outcome.

Air once was pure and was of such consistency that it was beyond the manipulation and control of humans. But since man discovered oil, manufactured automobiles and airplanes, built steel mills and other factories, etc., he has polluted the air.

The second source of life has an even sadder story to tell. FOOD for man was conceived by the great unknown Power that conceived Man, and Man and his Food were planned at the same time. Man tries to duplicate this natural food and to improve upon Nature, but has never succeeded. The food resulting from the *natural* process is complete; it is *just right*, and any change in it that is attempted by man makes it wrong.

The woeful story food has to tell us is this: after Nature bestows on Man an abundant variety of wholesome foods, the human hand processes it, combines it with unnatural materials, adulterates it, and then gives it a new name under the mocking title of "Pure Food." We attempt an impossible feat and when we fail we wonder why.

The body rebels against this abuse in the form of loss of hair, weakness of the eyes, colds, tonsillitis, indigestion, constipation, rheumatism, obesity, ulcers of the stomach, pneumonia, tuberculosis, piles, cancer, heart trouble, arthritis, and many other modern diseases. We ignore Food's plea to "Let me alone. How do you expect me to give you living cells when you destroy my vitality? I cannot do it . . . It cannot be done!"

Living matter cannot be made from dead matter. Take any seeds and cook them before planting, and they will not grow. We humans retort, "We live but once, and we might as well enjoy life." Now, do those who live to eat really enjoy life? Well, they do seemingly enjoy the few minutes they spend consuming their denatured food — but how about the hours that follow — the pressure of gas in the intestinal walls, the belching, the hours of nausea, the headaches, the fits of indigestion, the hours spent at the dentist and doctor? Does it pay?

Innocent and self-reliant Food exclaims: "Study me, look me over, give me the attention you give my unnatural and deceiving rivals. Try me out and I will reward you with just as good tastes . . . even better! . . . tastes which leave no evils behind in the form of coated tongue, stained teeth, decayed teeth, upset digestion, bad breath and disease.

The promise of natural food is — I will reward you with a clean body, a clean and peaceful mind, with an abundance of energy, with contentment, with efficiency, with health, with long life, with

A LIFE FREE FROM SUFFERING!

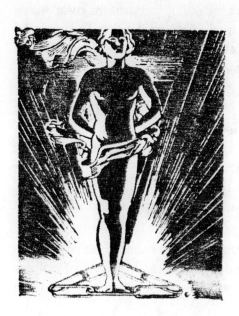

"In order to obtain optimum health, all Seven Essentials of Health should be adhered to."

— Dr. P. J. Welsh, in his work of the same title.

CHAPTER XIV

THE NATURAL WAY TO TREAT CONSTIPATION

There is scarcely an ailment which has been treated in so many ways and so unsuccessfully as constipation.

Constipation is one of the most prevalent ailments. Directly and indirectly it causes disease, discomfort and inefficiency. Constipation means much more than inability to move the bowels freely and regularly. It means the arrest of elimination, the clogging of the circulation of the blood, increased pressure on all nerves, and re-absorption of toxins and poisons which should be eliminated regularly.

Constipation pollutes the entire bloodstream, over-taxes the heart, affects the mind, and interferes with the normal function of every organ of the body. It is a destroyer of comfort, health, and happiness.

Many of the diseases of the human body are brought on by constipation. Therefore, in treating any ailment, it is important to begin the treatment with a cleansing of the colon with enemas, colemics or colonics, as suggested at the beginning of this book. This simple, safe procedure often brings immediate relief, yet it is so very often overlooked. Do remember this fact. It can at times mean the difference between life and death.

As a result of the crying need for the relief of constipation, many laxatives have come to our markets. Millions of dollars are spent each year by the many who are troubled with constipation.

By the use of these drugs, the bowels are forced to move; however, sooner or later, the drugs cause great damage to the delicate tissues of the digestive system.

These laxative drugs are weakening to the user because they not only drive out the morbid matter, but also take with them the intestinal secretions which are so necessary for bodily strength.

Besides damaging the body, these laxatives do not remove the cause of constipation. Therefore, they must be used continually.

The better and sensible way to combat constipation is to determine what are the causes of this ailment. Then, by removing these causes, we have a good chance to remedy the condition.

In the many years I have researched this problem, I have found the following to be the causes of constipation:

1. A faulty diet.
2. Lack of exercise.
3. Delay in answering "nature's call" to move the bowels.
4. Lack of sleep and rest.
5. Surgery and other traumas.
6. Obstruction in the colon.
7. Heredity

1. A FAULTY DIET

Of these seven causes of constipation, a faulty diet is the most important.

Never yet has anyone found constipation in any animal in its wild state. Domesticated animals, when fed our cooked and denatured foods, do suffer with constipation, but all animals away from the influence of our refined diet, never have constipation.

It is most important for those suffering with constipation *gradually* to include as many of the natural foods as possible. There are four classes of natural foods:

1. Raw, fresh, uncooked vegetables;
2. Raw, fresh, uncooked fruits;
3. Raw, fresh, uncooked and unprocessed nuts;
4. Seeds, grains, pulses, and sprouts (See Ch. V on Sprouting).

This gives us the following to choose from:

VEGETABLES

Cabbage	Endive	Radishes
Carrots	Leeks	Spinach
Cauliflower	Lettuce	Tomatoes
Celery	Parsley	Turnips
Corn	Peas	Watercress

FRUITS

Apple	Grapefruit	Papaya
Apricot	Grapes	Pear
Avocado	Honeydew melon	Persimmon
Bananas	Huckleberries	Pineapple
Blackberries	Lemon	Plum
Blueberries	Mango	Pomegranate
Cantaloupe	Muskmelon	Raspberries
Casaba melon	Nectarine	Sapotas
Cherries	Olives	Strawberries
Figs	Orange	Watermelon

NUTS

Almond	Chestnut	Pecan
Brazil	Coconut (fresh)	Pine nut
Cashew	Filbert	Walnut

SEEDS

Sesame (ground)	Sunflower	Pumpkin

WHOLE GRAINS

Wheat	Corn	Buckwheat
Rice	Millet	Oats, etc.

PULSES OR LEGUMES

Peas	Beans	Lentils

In order to function properly, the digestive and eliminating organs must have certain vitamins, organic minerals and enzymes. All of these are found in the natural foods and lacking in the processed, unnatural foods.

By this time, you can see that the same foods which serve to overcome constipation also rid the body of arthritis and other abnormal conditions of the organism.

Stubborn cases of constipation of long standing may need extra help, so here are a few suggestions:

1. Drink six glasses of water or fresh fruit juices each day — two in the morning, two at noon, and two during the afternoon.

2. Use two or three tablespoonsful of plain wheat or oat bran twice each day. The bran may be taken with water, fresh fruit juices, or fresh carrot juice. Also, it may be mixed with soaked prunes or figs. The bran may also be eaten with a bowl of fresh fruit and a little low-fat milk or soy or rice milk.

3. Use Psyllium seeds, flax seed, or Agar once a day. These three natural aids are obtainable in all health food stores, with directions for use on the package. These aids provide bulk as well as lubrication, which is so essential for normal bowel action.

4. Use "Sea-Klenz," a powder which comes from organic sea plants, especially kelp. (Call 800-350-LIFE to order.)

II. LACK OF EXERCISE

We will now consider the second requirement for the relief of constipation — exercise. The American people have really been spoiled when it comes to exercising. With the advent of the automobile and all the labor saving devices in our homes, most of our population gets far too little exercise.

By this time, every intelligent person should know that it is impossible to maintain good health without exercise. To fulfill this need, it is not necessary to go to a gymnasium or buy an assortment of gadgets. Ten minutes of simple setting-up exercises and a good walk each day will keep you fit if done *regularly*.

One of the best simple exercises is raising the arms overhead and bending forward as far as you can, comfortably. It is not necessary to touch the floor; just bend over as far as you can. Begin with a few bends and gradually increase the number. By doing them rapidly, it takes only a few minutes.

Another good simple one is to hold on to a chair with one hand and kick up, first one foot, then the other.

These plus two or three other simple exercises you can think of, will do a lot for your circulation and muscular system. The trick is to make it a habit, and then it will not be a hardship.

In addition, it is very important to take a good walk each day in the cool of the day, and *not* in the hot sunshine.

One of the reasons why the American people are the most constipated people in the world is because they do so little walking. The ever increasing use of automobiles and elevators, the great desire to save time and the horribly constructed shoes* are three reasons why the American people neglect to walk.

---

*In the U.S., fashion prevails over comfort in women's shoes.

In a recent survey by the U.S.C. School of Medicine and the American Orthopaedic Foot and Ankle Society, 88% of women were wearing shoes smaller than their feet; 80% said that their feet hurt. There is a connection.

Dr. Carol Frey of U.S.C. said, "Most cases of bunions, hammertoes, corns and calluses in women are directly related to the shoes they wear. They need to start wearing shoes that fit." Frey, the study's principal investigator, joined the society's women's footwear committee in interviewing 356 women ages 20 to 60. The women were asked to bring a "typical fashion shoe" from their wardrobe to the researchers, who traced the shoes and the women's feet. When the tracings were measured, researchers found the great majority of shoes were smaller than the great majority of feet. In many cases, the feet were far wider than the "fashion" shoes. Frey notes that some companies do not make shoes in the "C" width many women need.

Note by Dr. Leonardo: This is not a recent trend. When I was a girl, my wide feet (at least C's) were squeezed into shoes that were B's. A bunion developed on the wider foot. Much later, I realized that I had to do something, and that was to either wear athletic shoes much of the time, or shop at special stores with wide shoes for women. Twice I found shoes I could wear in men's shoe stores.

Before reading this article (from *The Los Angeles Times*), I suspected this was true, both from my own experience, and also from looking at women's feet, often obviously squeezed into a shoe too narrow for them. That is also why women often slip off their pumps whenever they can. High heels are another fashion monstrosity, very harmful to the foot's bone structure.

Men will not tolerate such a condition; they won't wear shoes that don't fit, and men's fashion does not demand that they do so.

It is impossible to cure constipation without walking. Trying to overcome constipation without walking is like trying to learn to swim without going into the water. It cannot be done.

Walking is the best and most natural exercise there is. This simple exercise is absolutely essential for the cure of constipation, and the more one walks the sooner will the cure by accomplished. As soon as you begin to walk constipation begins to go — providing, of course, that the other requirements are adhered to, explained in this chapter.

The motion of walking causes every one of the internal and digestive organs to be massaged and gently stimulates their function. It increases the peristaltic action of the entire intestinal tract, and causes the food to pass through the intestinal tract with dispatch, so that the residue reaches the rectum in a copious, moist and lubricated form. In that way it sends a very pronounced and definite impulse to the nerves of the colon and rectum, with the result that the individual is obliged to stop and relieve himself of this residue.

If, however, the individual does not walk and leads a sedentary life, the food does not travel through the digestive tract in the right length of time. Its progress is delayed, and by the time it reaches the rectum, all the water has been absorbed, and the residue is in the form of a dry, sticky mass hard to expel.

Again, when the individual neglects this essential of walking, the residue reaches the colon in small quantities, and therefore the impulse to the nerves in the colon is not pronounced, with the result that the call to relieve the bowels is overlooked. These small quantities then gradually accumulate without any further impulses, and the result is that this toxic matter remains there for days, infecting, irritating and polluting the entire system, and causing many unsuspected disturbances.

Walking induces deep breathing. Deep breathing causes the diaphragm to move more freely with each breath, and this gentle and continuous movement of the diaphragm massages the digestive and other organs, and in that way increases and improves their function of digesting and lubricating the residue. Walking will not only help to cure your constipation, but will also strengthen and improve every part of your body.

It is distressing, annoying and virtually impossible to enjoy walking with the ordinary shoe, so obtain an extremely comfortable shoe, and walk at every opportunity you have.

If possible, walk in the country away from the noise, dirt, gas fumes and traffic. Take off as many unnecessary clothes as possible and get into the stride of this simple but marvelous health restorer, walking.

Running, jumping, golf, tennis, ball playing, swimming, dancing, and mountain climbing — all the natural forms of exercise and recreation are very beneficial. You will soon find out that exercising is something that will pay you big dividends in health and happiness.

The occupation of an individual has a direct bearing upon the action of the bowels. Those who do physical work out of doors suffer much less with constipation than indoor sedentary workers. If there is any choice in the matter of occupation, I cannot urge you too strongly to choose the physical outdoor work.

Before leaving this subject, let us consider the few unfortunate ones who are confined and cannot walk. Such persons should confine themselves to the vegetable and fruit juice diet until they are able to walk. By adhering to this diet they will benefit in two ways. They will avoid constipation and also bring about a most rapid recovery from their other ailment which hinders them from walking.

But you who are blessed with a good pair of legs and feet should take advantage of this simple, easy, convenient, costless yet priceless health restorer — walking. Women! Throw off your tight, stiff, high heeled shoes — get the most comfortable shoe you can buy and at every opportunity, get out of doors and walk. Walk at a good rapid pace. Try to walk after each meal. Walk to and from business, if possible. On Sundays and holidays get out into the mountains, in the woods or on the beach, away from those deadly gasoline fumes. Walk, run, jump, and give your body a chance to absorb all the wonderful vitalic forces of Nature. It will help you cure constipation, as well as rejuvenate your entire body. Try it without fail!

III. NOT ANSWERING NATURE'S CALL PROMPTLY

In these days of strife and stress we are so busy trying to accomplish more than we should that we try to squeeze 48 hours of work into 24. Instead of trying to do this by increasing our efficiency through a healthy and smooth-running body and mind, we are doing just the reverse.

In our great rush and excitement, we overlook every essential of health. We overlook every one of the natural requirements for well being. We rush to the restaurant, gulp down anything handed out by the waiter behind the counter, rush back and forth under a nerve racking strain which makes normal digestion and elimination impossible.

Most people do not even take the necessary time to answer nature's call to move the bowels. When the call is overlooked, constipation will result. This mad rush and neglect to stop, rest and answer the call of nature is one of the definite causes of constipation, and should be remedied at once if you wish results. The habit of moving the bowels should be a habit of rest as well as one of comfort.

The hour of eating is a very sacred time of the day, for it is then that you are building the human temple. First, throw off the rushing attitude. Become calm and peaceful. Take off your business clothes if possible. They are often filled with negative vibrations and unpleasant associations. Make yourself as comfortable as possible, away from all distressing and annoying surroundings. Wash your hands, face and body if possible, and then quietly sit down not to talk business, but to build your human temple, the greatest and most worthy mechanism every conceived.

Sit down if possible in your own private chamber, or better still in the sunshine, and enjoy satisfying a hungry appetite — an appetite which will appreciate the remarkable flavors of the natural foods.

Eat these natural foods peacefully, and to your heart's content. After each meal take time to attend to your bowel movement. This should not be hurried, forced or strained. Upon the slightest impulse or notification, go without delay to the toilet with some piece of interesting reading matter. Sit down on the toilet seat and bend over so that the shoulders are touching the knees. Place the reading matter on the floor between your feet, and forget about moving the bowels.

Now, after you have assumed this bent position with the shoulders touching the knees (this position is very important) then begin to do what is known as abdominal breathing. When you inhale take the air in as if it were going into your stomach and not into the chest. Keep the mouth closed and do this abdominal breathing and then take your mind off this act by reading your book or magazine which should be on the floor between your feet. In a few moments you will have a natural bowel movement.

It is wrong to strain and force a bowel movement. As a rule those suffering with constipation are so bent on moving the bowels that they begin to strain as soon as they are seated on the toilet. This contracts the muscles of the anus and actually prevents a complete movement with the result that even if a movement is accomplished it is incomplete and never satisfactory. I cannot stress too much the importance of learning this technique of moving the bowels without straining. Again, let me give you the steps of this important act.

1.   Answer Nature's call to move the bowels as soon as possible.

2.   Seated on the toilet, bend over until the knees are touching the shoulder.

3.   Relax and begin abdominal breathing.

4.   Divert the attention by reading some interesting matter placed on the floor between the feet.

5.   Clasp your hands behind your legs.

If you have carried out the requirements mentioned throughout this work you will be rewarded with a natural bowel movement that will surprise and please you.

The squatting position is the natural and best way to help the bowels move, but Western toilets are designed too high to do this. That is why I have given you the preceding instructions, to take the place of squatting. You can help your bowels move naturally by placing a low stool in front of the toilet bowl and squatting on this stool.

IV. INSUFFICIENT SLEEP

The fourth requirement for overcoming constipation is sufficient sleep and rest.

Sleep is the great restorer — the re-builder. During the day, especially under our complex living conditions, the body is being torn down and worn out. It is during sleep that most of the rebuilding takes place. It stands to reason that if we expect to rebuild and strengthen the intestinal tract, we must give the body sufficient sleep to do so. Different individuals require varying amounts of sleep, but very few can do their bodies justice on fewer than eight hours. During the day the body is in an upright position with a constant expenditure of energy to support the various functions of the organs, as well as the stress that arises frequently. During sleep, each organ and the body as a whole has the greatest opportunity to perform its various functions including digestion and elimination with the least expenditure of energy.

In observing patients who were inclined toward constipation, I have noticed time and again that if these patients did not get their full quota of sleep, they had difficulty in moving their bowels.

I have written extensively on the subject of sleep in my work *The Seven Essentials of Health,* so I will not attempt to cover the same ground here. However, let me advise you who are serious in overcoming constipation to get to bed early, so that you will get all the sleep you require.

It is best not to drink much water or other liquids before retiring, for it may be the cause of disturbing your sleep, by the necessity of urinating. However, when you are in bed, if you get the impulse to either urinate or move the bowels, DON'T PUT IT OFF, but get right up and do so. Then return to bed; you will feel much better and sleep more soundly. Remember never to put off these important duties of emptying either the bladder or the bowels.

V. SURGERY AND OTHER TRAUMAS

It often happens that during surgery, the nerves and muscles controlling the function of the bowels are damaged. As a result, the patient is unable to have a natural bowel movement. This is unfortunate, and at times frustrating.

But fortunately, we have a way of overcoming this disadvantage, and that is the use of the enema, which in such cases is truly a "godsend."

The taking of an enema is a simple procedure, yet there are some pointers which will be helpful to those who are not acquainted with this procedure. It is therefore advisable to read the material on the "Cleansing Process" in Chapter II.

In some cases where the patient has had an automobile accident, the same condition as above results, when the eliminating organs are damaged. In such cases, also, the patient will have to resort to the enema.

VI. OBSTRUCTION IN THE LUMEN (opening) OF THE COLON

Occasionally (fortunately, not often) the colon is partially or completely closed by an abnormal growth or tumor.

In such cases, the obstruction must be removed, either with surgery or by fasting and other natural methods.

VII. HEREDITY

Finally, we come to the seventh and last of the causes of constipation, and that is Heredity. By that we mean there are certain tendencies each of us is born with, tendencies we inherit from our parents.

Some persons are born with a tendency for a thick growth of hair, while others are born with a tendency for a scanty crop of hair, and early baldness.

The same is true of teeth. Some inherit a fine set of teeth, and others, poor, irregular teeth. And so it is with the action of the bowels. Some of us inherit healthy, *active* bowels, and others sluggish bowels.

If you have inherited active bowels, you are fortunate, and should have no trouble with constipation. But if you inherited sluggish bowels, then you will have to give special attention to that function of your body. You will be obliged to resort to every aid available to insure adequate elimination of the waste products constantly being deposited in the colon. In such cases, the information I have given you in this chapter will be of great benefit, and you should study the advice carefully, and try to follow the suggestions as faithfully as possible.

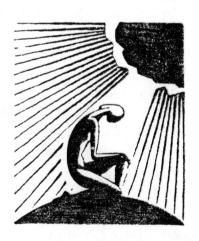

"Nature never did betray
The heart that loved her."

William Wordsworth

CHAPTER XV

THE VALUE OF THINGS

by

Benjamin Franklin

When I was a child seven years old, my friends on a holiday filled my pocket with coppers. I went directly to a shop where they sold toys for children, and being charmed with the sound of a whistle that I met by the way in the hands of another boy, I voluntarily offered and gave all my money for one. I then ran home and went whistling all over the house, much pleased with my whistle, but disturbing all the family.

My brothers and sisters and cousins, understanding the bargain I had made, told me I had given four times as much for it as it was worth; put me in mind what good things I might have bought with the rest of the money; and laughed at me so much for my folly that I cried with vexation; and the reflection gave me more chagrin than the whistle gave me pleasure.

This, however, was afterwards of use to me, the impression continuing on my mind; so that often when I was tempted to buy some unnecessary thing, I said to myself, "Don't give too much for the whistle," and I saved my money.

As I grew up, came into the world, and observed the actions of men, I thought I met with many, very many, who gave too much for the whistle.

When I saw one too ambitious of court favor, sacrificing his time in attendance on levees — his repose, his liberty, his virtue, and perhaps his friends, to attain it — I have said to myself, "This man gives too much for his whistle."

When I saw another, fond of popularity, constantly employing himself in political bustles, neglecting his own affairs, and ruining them by that neglect, "He pays indeed," said I, "too much for his whistle."

If I knew a miser who gave up every kind of comfortable living, all the pleasure of doing good for others, all the esteem of his fellow citizens, and the joys of benevolent friendship, for the sake of accumulating wealth, "Poor man," said I, "you pay too much for your whistle."

When I met with a man of pleasure, sacrificing every laudable improvement of the mind or of his fortune to mere corporeal sensations, and ruining his health in their pursuit, "Mistaken man," said I, "You are providing pain for yourself instead of pleasure; and give too much for your whistle."

If I see one fond of appearance, or fine clothes, fine houses, fine furniture, fine equipages, all above his fortune, for which he contracts debts and ends his career in a prison, "Alas!" say I, "he has paid dear for his whistle."

In short, I conceive that a great part of the miseries of mankind are brought upon them by the false estimates they have made of the value of things, and by their giving too much for their whistles. (The end of Ben Franklin's story.)

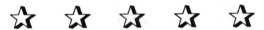

Why have we included the story of the whistle, or "The Value of Things" in this arthritis manual?

The reason is because some of our readers may be so addicted to unnatural foods that they would rather continue indulging in them as a result, suffer constant pain and often early death. To them we would say, "Are you paying too much for your whistle?"

The tongue is a small member of the body, but capable of causing great trouble, both in erroneous talking and in titillating the taste buds. Many persons consider only taste and totally disregard the harmfulness of certain foods and ingredients. Instead of having the mind in control, the tongue is in control.

So, consider: Are you "paying too much for your whistle" when you eat foods that on the one hand give you momentary pleasure, but on the other give you permanent pain? Isn't the price you pay with pain too great? The decision is yours.

☆ ☆ ☆ ☆ ☆

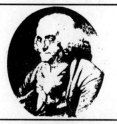
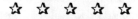
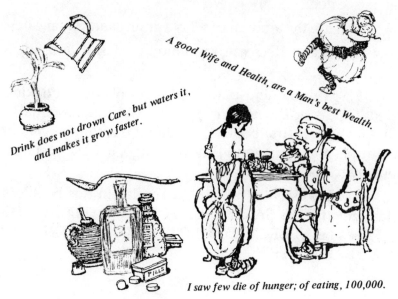

DIETARY GOALS FOR THE UNITED STATES

In 1968, the U.S. government realized that the American people were hurting their health as a result of harmful dietary habits, so it ordered a thorough investigation of this important problem. The Senate set up the Select Committee on Nutrition and Human Needs, with Senator George McGovern as Chairman.

Many prominent scientists and nutritionists were enlisted to help this committee with this project. Over a period of nine years, numerous hearings were held and testimonies recorded. Finally, after extensive staff studies of the material, the Committee's conclusions were formulated. They included the following recommendations for changes in the diet of Americans:*

* The complete Senate report (83 pages) can be obtained from the Superintendent of Documents, U.S. Printing Office, Washington, D.C. 20402. Ask for "Dietary Goals for the U.S.," second edition, Stock No. 052-070-04376-8.

1. Reduce the intake of fat, especially animal fats.

2. Increase the amounts of fresh fruit and fresh vegetables eaten.

3. Increase the amount of whole grains and cereal eaten.

4. Drastically decrease the amount of salt and sugar eaten.

In 1929, I wrote and published a set of seven booklets entitled *The Seven Essentials of Health*. The first essential is Fresh Air. In this first booklet, I pointed out the dangers of air pollution and smog (and fifty years ago, it was much less serious than it is today).

The second essential is Natural Foods. In this booklet I recommended THE SAME DIET FORMULATED BY THE U.S. SENATE SELECT COMMITTEE ON NUTRITION FORTY YEARS LATER!

CHOLESTEROL IN A NUTSHELL

The health news of the '90s includes much on cholesterol. While it can become somewhat technical, there are simple facts easy to remember — namely, which foods have a high content of harmful cholesterol, and which foods have none. Here is a simple chart:

Cholesterol Content
(In milligrams, per 100 gram portion)

Animal Foods		Plant Foods	
Eggs, whole	550	All grains	0
Kidney, beef	375	Vegetables	0
Liver	300	Nuts	0
Butter	250	Seeds	0
Oysters	200	Fruits	0
Cream Cheese	120	Legumes	0
Lard	95	Vegetable Oils	0
Beefsteak	70		
Pork	70		
Chicken	60		
Ice Cream	45		

Now, you can draw your own conclusions as to which foods you wish to emphasize in your diet, for better health and normal weight.

In addition to the cholesterol in meat products, there are other unhealthful aspects. Meat is capable of producing cancer-causing agents in the colon. In contrast, a vegetarian diet can reduce the incidence of cancer of the colon by 40%. Meat can contain carcinogenic substances.

Animals are dosed regularly with antibiotics. So, even people who do not get medical antibiotics, are getting them via the meat they eat. Food poisoning is very common; most of it is meat and poultry-related.

Meat production is having a catastrophic effect, particularly in the Third World. To satisfy the insatiable meat demands of the West, 40% of the world's cereal harvest goes to feed livestock. It actually takes ten pounds of grain to produce just one pound of beef. At least ten times as many people can be supported on a vegetarian diet, yet at any time 500 million people throughout the world are severely malnourished.

CHAPTER XVI

AN OUTSTANDING CASE

One of the most outstanding cases and one of the most memorable persons I ever encountered in my career of over fifty years of practice was a nurse named Rebecca.

After the birth of her first child she became sick and developed one ailment after another. In spite of the treatments she received from some of the most renowned doctors and specialists of the day, she became worse and worse until all hope of recovery was gone. Her last doctor, who had heard of my work in preventive dentistry, sent her to me to have her teeth extracted — with the hope that this would at least help rid her of arthritis. She dreaded losing her teeth, but was willing to do anything to become free from her constant pain.

During our first appointment she gave me her complete history. Her story was a woeful one — a long list of disappointing treatments and unsuccessful surgery — and in the end a grossly overweight body that was constantly harassed by the aches and pains of arthritis.

After X-raying her teeth, I found they were in good shape, in spite of the fact that she had pyorrhea. Instead of extracting her teeth, I changed her diet! I had learned that in treating conditions of mouth the natural way, instead of with drugs, one must treat the body as a whole — and as a result, when the mouth is healed, the other parts of the body benefit also. In holistic healing, we use constitutional methods as well as local ones.

I explained to Rebecca that she, being a medical nurse, had been trained along medical lines and had depended upon drugs and surgery for help to recover from sickness. I explained that our methods are entirely different in that we use no drugs and no surgery. Instead, we use natural methods, adopting and following the natural laws of health, which involve nutrition, exercise, rest, fresh air, water, sunshine, and positive thinking.

I explained how the human body has a wonderful ability to heal itself, but that in order to do so, it must have no interference. In other words, if we want Nature to heal our body we have to cooperate by obeying the strict laws of Nature. I explained how if we breathe polluted air, eat denatured and devitalized foods, do not get proper rest, do not observe the laws of hygiene by being clean internally as well as externally, etc., we cannot expect good health. I impressed upon her the fact that there are certain definite, natural requirements which have to be fulfilled — that if we do our part, Nature will do Hers, and the results will be good.

These principles of natural healing were new to Rebecca. She had never heard of such a simple, natural way of healing the human body. She was dazed, but I could see that she was intensely interested and very receptive.

When I was all through I paused and said, "So, you see, Rebecca, your recovery from your ailments will depend upon how well you will heed the laws of Nature and how conscientiously you will apply them. I will do all I can to show you the way, but you will have to do your part."

I then arose to dismiss her. She stood up, clasped both my hands, and with the utmost sincerity assured me that she would follow all my instructions carefully. And this she certainly did.

She went home, threw out all of the white sugar, white flour, and salt, then disposed of all the canned goods in her house. She refilled her refrigerator and cupboards with fresh fruits, fresh vegetables, honey, nuts, and whole grains. She began to take daily walks and to take sun baths.

In all my fifty years' experience I have never seen a patient make such a radical change in so short a time, and with such good results. She not only changed her own mode of living, but that of her husband and children. It was not too long before Rebecca was a new woman. Her aches and pains were gone — and so was her excess weight. She became as slender as a young girl. Her husband's weight also became normal and his health was restored, too. Her hope and confidence returned — and for all that she was most thankful. She expressed radiant health.

Rebecca never missed an opportunity to show her gratitude. She was so enthusiastic about her new knowledge of natural living that whenever she heard of a friend or neighbor who was ailing she would go to him or her and nurse the patient back to health — without any remuneration! She was one who really lived for others instead of for herself. If ever an angel walked on this planet, Rebecca was such a one. She lived a long time — outliving all the doctors who had given her up to die.

The following is a letter Rebecca wrote me four years after her first visit. She had learned I was writing my course on *The Seven Essentials of Health* and this inspired her to write me this letter of gratitude.

Dear Dr. Welsh:

I am sending you this letter so that those who are not yet acquainted with your work may be influenced to grasp this opportunity of getting your course, which will open their eyes to the true principles of health the way it did for me.

I was a trained nurse at the Montefiore Hospital in New York, and all went well until I married and gave birth to my first child. After my confinement, I felt myself getting weaker and weaker, and soon found myself tortured with one ailment after another — constipation, headaches, burning pains in my feet, sagging of abdominal organs, abscesses of the breast, pyorrhea and other very depressing symptoms.

Being a nurse by profession, I trusted the medical profession. I had a very prominent doctor operate on my abdominal organs, but after the operation I felt worse. I then visited a number of doctors. However, each day I felt myself slipping until I was utterly discouraged and ready to give it all up. I then telephoned my last doctor to tell him I was through and would take no more treatments. He pleaded with me not to give up and urged me to get in touch with you.

I will never forget how wonderfully you, Dr. Welsh, explained the principles underlying life, and how to live in health and happiness — all so simple that I felt dazed with unbelief.

My husband, who was suffering with sinus trouble, heartburn, headaches, rheumatism and weighed over 200 pounds, then became interested.

It is now four years since we adopted your plan. Chaos, despair and sickness have given way to peace, happiness and perfect health. My husband is more successful and efficient than he ever was. Our children are a wonder in health and cleverness, and for all of these blessings we are thanking you, Dr. Welsh, for you led us out of the desert and into the promised land of Natural Living.

Your forever faithful friend,

(signed) Rebecca Szainman

But the story does not end here. At the time Rebecca came to me she had a chubby, smiling baby girl named Deborah. Naturally, this child was brought up in the new mode of living her mother and father had adopted.

After Deborah grew up she met and married Professor Edmond Bordeaux Szekely, a noted scholar and author of many books. Together they founded *Rancho La Puerta*, one of the largest and most famous health resorts in America. Later Deborah founded the world-renowned health spa, *The Golden Door*, in Escondido, California. The *Golden Door* has brought health and rejuvenation to many prominent persons, including movie stars.

Rancho La Puerta, located in Tecate, Mexico, is also doing a marvelous job bringing health and relaxation to the many who come and return again and again for rest, recreation and improved health.

Today Deborah Szekely is a prominent, dynamic person, actively spreading the gospel of good health throughout the nation.

In 1976 she received the annual award from the California Business Administration: "Person of the Year." She is the first woman ever to be so honored. She is the author of a book, *Secrets of The Golden Door*.

It is a happy thought to know that the seeds I planted over fifty years ago are bearing such good fruit today.

Dr. Edmond Bordeaux Szekely, Deborah's husband, was a scholar and author. His discovery and translation of an important document in the Vatican Archives resulted in his publication of *The Essene Gospel of Peace*, believed to be the lost words of Jesus on food and diet. In spiritual and poetic language, it presents the humane diet of Jesus, the disciples and the Essenes of his day. Over one million copies have been sold, and it has appeared in 26 languages. Here is a great treasure, available from Tree of Life Publications ($2.00 postpaid.)

I, Dr. Leonardo, studied the Essene teachings with Dr. Edmond B. Szekely during five years when he was teaching in San Diego, California.

CHAPTER XVII

HISTORY REPEATS ITSELF

Many years ago, the dental profession knew nothing about nutrition. Patients were told and dental students were taught that the way to prevent caries (tooth decay) was to merely keep the teeth clean. Not a single word about nutrition! It was then that I made extensive tests of this theory on many of my patients' teeth and on my own teeth, and found that it did not work. At the time, I was deeply involved in the study of nutrition, so I decided to apply the principles of nutrition for the prevention of tooth decay. After several years of research along this line, I was convinced that nutrition is of prime importance in the prevention of tooth decay.

Then, in 1925, the Chicago Dental Society conducted an "Oral Hygiene Week." To obtain material to be broadcast during that week, they announced a contest. They invited all the dentists in the nation to submit essays, the winners to be broadcast over the radio networks.

I, a young dentist with a new practice, submitted an essay in which I stated that I had tested the then-prevalent theory that "A clean tooth will not decay," and found IT WAS NOT SO! That nutrition had to be considered also.

At the conclusion of the contest, I was chosen as one of the seven winners, and received an award for my revolutionary finding. (See the Chicago Dental Society letter reproduced in Chapter I.)

Now, many years later, it is common knowledge that sugar harms the teeth and that nutrition has a great deal to do with dental health.

NOW THE MEDICAL PROFESSION IS MAKING THE SAME MISTAKE ABOUT BODY ILLNESSES (that nutrition has nothing to do with them) THAT THE DENTAL PROFESSION MADE IN THE 1920's (about nutrition having nothing to do with dental health)! This is because during the long medical training of doctors, there is much instruction in the use of drugs and surgery, but very little, if anything, is taught about nutrition!

There is a common phrase, "We are what we eat," but this truth has not yet penetrated medical studies.

THE DOCTORS ARE TELLING THEIR PATIENTS THAT NUTRITION HAS NOTHING TO DO WITH ARTHRITIS. AGAIN, I SAY THEY ARE WRONG. I HAVE THE PROOF, and sooner or later, they will have to reverse themselves. The details of this important controversy is in this book.

Every sufferer from arthritis should read the facts in this book. The first five editions have helped many persons, and given us a feedback — substantial evidence on results that are being obtained, proving that this plan really works. You hold in your hands a copy of the sixth edition.

CHAPTER XVIII

HEALTH CAPSULES

We are constantly researching the subject of arthritis and nutrition, and with each new edition, we add information that we have learned. In this way, we bring the very latest to our readers.

LIGHT EXERCISE A GREAT HELP

We have written about walking in this book. Scientific studies now show that any physical activity (kind and amount) is beneficial for people who are sedentary. A landmark study by Stanford researcher Ralph S. Pfaffenbarger, Jr., M.D., with 12,000 men (Harvard alumni) involved, showed that the death rate decreased about 21% among previously sedentary men who became moderately active in various sports during middle age or later, and that the death rate is lower among people who are more fit. The *Journal of the American Medical Association,* in an accompanying editorial, stated that "even modest improvement in fitness level among the most unfit confers a substantial health benefit."

So, get out and walk, or swim, or bicycle—whatever you like to do and can do. Instead of being a "couch potato," you can watch some television while on your stationary bicycle, rebounder, or other indoor exercise equipment.

EATING TIPS

Years ago, a man named Fletcher recommended that people chew each mouthful thirty times before swallowing; the word "fletcherize" arose from this practice. That may seem strange to you, but it is "food for thought." Here are some valuable eating tips, for better digestion and health.

• During meals, eat small bites of food; chew until the food is liquefied and then swallow. Since it takes up to twenty minutes for your brain to get the message that the body is full, eating slowly will help prevent overeating.

• Eating is a social event in most cases, instead of merely a solo event for nourishment purposes. This creates a problem; the mouth cannot talk and chew well at the same time. The talker is swallowing unchewed food. People won't stop socializing while eating, but the solution can be taking your time when eating. As you take one bite, put your fork down. You can change your eating habits. Try to alternate chewing/swallowing with talking.

• While eating, don't drink water with the meal because it dilutes the hydrochloric acid in the stomach which is needed to break down food. Water or other drinks should be drunk at least thirty minutes before meals or two hours after.

• The most healthful liquids are pure water, herbal tea, organic vegetable juices (preferably freshly squeezed at home), and soups. Undesirable liquids, from a health standpoint, are: traditional (black or green) tea, sodas, coffee, cocoa, bottled or canned drinks or fruit juice. It is better to eat the whole orange (the white part gives us the valuable riboflavinoids), rather than juicing it, which fragments it.

• Don't feel compelled to eat everything on your plate. When you get through eating, you should never feel overstuffed. Your appestat tells you when to eat, and when to stop.

• Don't flavor your food with salt. Many foods naturally contain sodium and by shaking salt onto our food, the chance for retaining water and increasing our blood pressure is increased, as well as the development of arthritis.

• Eating several small meals a day (five or six) works better for the body than eating three large ones. This is because your blood sugar levels are maintained and thus the "yo-yo" effect is avoided (extreme hunger, then stuffing oneself).

• Diets high in fibrous foods, such as whole grains, vegetables and fruits, will also help aid in weight loss because they add food value without adding many calories. These foods are also filling because we must chew them, which makes us feel more satisfied with less food. We give our gums exercise, and much chewing gives the saliva, with its enzymes, an opportunity to act on the food. The first step in digestion takes place in the mouth. Remember, the stomach has no teeth, so watch swallowing pieces of food that have not been chewed well.

AGAIN, THE AMAZING APPLE

Every child has heard the old adage, "An apple a day keeps the doctor away." Folk wisdom and modern science agree. We have already written about the apple, elsewhere, but here bring you a mention of a new scientific study.

Researchers at the University of Texas Health Science Center in San Antonio say that pectin, as found in apples, can both reduce the incidence of colon cancer and lower blood cholesterol levels by 27 to 30 %.

They studied the effects of cellulose (a vegetable fiber) on colon health, and noted that cellulose fiber can lower the incidence of colon cancer, but could not lower levels of cholesterol. When they tested pectin, however, they were successful in lowering both. They added that "100% of pectin is digested, whereas cellulose is not digested at all." The researchers suspect that pectin and cellulose halt the progression of cancer by interfering with carcinogens that harm genetic material within cells.

BETA-CAROTENE TO THE RESCUE IN HEART DISEASE

It was in the 1970's that the first announcement was made that in countries where diets are rich in beta-carotene, the incidence of cancer is very low. The National Cancer

Institute is convinced of the health potential of beta-carotene foods.

You should eat lots of fruits and vegetables, especially the orange, yellow, and leafy green kinds, for protection.

The authors of this book recommend that you eat these fruits and vegetables in the raw state, as much as possible. Cooking destroys the valuable enzymes in foods. And freshly-squeezed orange and carrot juice has more value than previously prepared juices.

A recent finding showed that those persons taking beta-carotene supplements had 40% fewer heart attacks than those who were taking an inactive placebo. In a separate study at Johns Hopkins University, there were almost 50% fewer heart disease cases in a group of people with the highest levels of beta-carotene, compared to the group with the lowest levels.

FORTUNES SPENT NEEDLESSLY

San Francisco (UPI) — Americans have become pill-popping, chronic complainers who spend a fortune making needless trips to the doctor's office, according to a Stanford University researcher.

Dr. James F. Fries said that individuals should look to the historic self-reliance of America's pioneers, instead of reaching for a pill every time something ails them.

He recommends that people practice their own preventive medicine by adopting healthful habits and setting health goals. (Authors' note: That is the theme of our book.)

DOCTOR SAYS NAPPING IS GOOD

Chicago (UPI) — Napping is good for you. Done properly, research indicates, it improves business performance, increases a feeling of well-being and reduces anxiety.

Habitual nappers don't lie awake at nights because they nap during the day. The nap is a restorative, the researchers said. It enables the napper to fall asleep more easily at night and sleep more soundly.

EXERCISING ON YOUR VACATION

Don't let your exercise schedule take a back seat to your vacation and travel. Gear your workouts to the locale. And above all, keep it easy, and you'll stick to your schedule.

CAN CHOCOLATE TURN ONE INTO A CRIMINAL?

(Some Experts Say So)

Washington: *The Wall Street Journal* — Society is always debating the causes of crime. The discussion generally centers around social, hereditary and economic factors. But lately more attention is being given to a biological source of anti-social behavior: the food people eat.

An increasing number of scientists and physicians are concluding that malnutrition, food allergies and other nutritional deficiencies can set off aggressive and mind-warping behavior leading to criminal acts. (We have already written about this in our book.)

SOFT DRINKS

The average American drank the equivalent of more than 550 cans of soft drinks during the year 1990. Unless these were diet drinks, that adds up to over 83,000 empty calories per person. Unless these calories were counteracted by increased exercise, they could result in a weight gain of almost 24 pounds a year.

If only Americans could resist the ubiquitous advertising for such products, and realize they are being influenced to buy and use harmful foods and non-foods!

BREADS

There are many kinds of bread: the white breads in our supermarkets are abominable.

The better breads in the health food stores are the organic, whole wheat breads, the sprouted wheat breads, and the low-sodium (no salt added) breads.

If possible, bake your own, and instead of salt, use onion and caraway seeds for flavor.

Some of the bakers have the crazy notion that wheat berries are good in breads. The fact is that after baking, these wheat berries become as hard as rocks; they can break your teeth, and wreck your digestive organs. Wheat berries are good for birds, but not for humans, unless soaked and sprouted.

We personally use very little bread, and never fresh bread. The fresh bread is fattening and mucus-forming; but when thoroughly toasted and re-baked under the broiler, instead of in the toaster, the bread is easier to digest and is not mucus-forming and fattening. (We realize we are asking you to give up sandwiches. Most sandwich combinations are poor.) If this toasted bread is too hard for you, soften with a liquid, such as vegetable broth.

Better than bread are the sliced, toasted potatoes, the recipe for which you will find in Chapter IV.

CONCERNING ORGANIC FOODS

The fact that a food is organic does not guarantee the quality. Fruits should be tree-ripened, and naturally sweet, especially berries, cherries and peaches. Fruit that is picked too soon does not have the nourishment of tree-ripened fruit. Hard, unripe fruit is sour; one can keep it in a dark cupboard until soft and edible, but it still will not be like tree-ripened fruit.

DAIRY PRODUCTS

Many people are using too large a quantity of dairy products. As a result, they develop a great deal of sickness. The worst of the dairy products is store cheese. These cheeses are concentrated, mucus-forming foods, which clog the body, especially the sinuses, the nose, throat and respiratory organs, causing colds, coughs, bronchitis and pneumonia. They cause excess cholesterol and heart trouble. In addition, these processed cheeses cause constipation and overweight.

The salt, artificial colorings and preservatives found in most cheeses, are very bad for arthritis. We recommend the home-made buttermilk cheese, the recipe for which you will find in this book. Also acceptable is the soy-based cheese found in health food stores.

Butter, whole milk and eggs should be used in moderation, if at all. The ordinary salted butter is one cause of arthritis and heart trouble, as well as high blood pressure. If butter is used, it should be unsalted and used sparingly.

When possible, use avocado instead of butter. Avocado is a natural fat which will not clog the system, and will not cause overweight. Believe it or not, a pound of avocados will put on less weight than one ounce of butter!

Milk should be certified, raw, low-fat or non-fat. If it is used as a drink, it is a good idea to mix it half-and-half with fresh carrot juice. Milk is useful in cases of ulcers of the stomach. In such cases, the low-fat and certified raw, non-fat milk are better than whole milk.

Olive oil also is very helpful in ulcer cases. Use a tablespoonful three or four times a day.

MARGARINE

This artificial food should not be used, because it contains ingredients that do not belong in the human diet. However, a soy-based margarine is now available in health food stores.

YOGURT

This dairy food has become very popular, and used extensively by health-minded persons. However, most brands contain gelatin (which comes from the bones of animals), and artificial flavorings. The base is pasteurized milk, to which a culture has been added. Sometimes, sugar substitutes are added, harmful to the body.

You can make your own yogurt; it is a very simple process. Health food stores carry yogurt makers, which come with complete instructions. You can then add any of the pure, natural fruits for flavoring, and honey, if you wish.

AN ADDED WORD ABOUT SWEET CORN

When you are buying corn on the cob, if you see that all the ears are perfect, the chances are that the corn has been treated with a chemical pesticide. So, in buying corn, be suspicious when all the ears are perfect, and instead welcome an occasional worm. You will find that the corn which has not been chemically treated will taste much better and is more enjoyable. It is healthful, too.

The supermarkets seldom carry organic produce. Seek out other sources.

SALADS AND GREENS

Salads are very important in the diet, and should be eaten *every day*.

Greens are nutritious, since plant leaves and stems are basic makers of the nutrients that all animals subsist on.

Greens are low in calories and sodium and are fat-free.

Many varieties, especially kale, collards, and others in the cabbage family are rich in beta carotene.

They are good sources of iron, calcium, and other minerals and fiber.

In general, the darker the leaves, the more nutritious. For example, romaine lettuce has six times more Vitamin C and eight times more Beta Carotene than iceberg lettuce.

Many salads contain large chunks of raw vegetables, that require too much chewing. Most people do not take the time to chew and chew, so they swallow the chunks of salad ingredients, which pass through the digestive tract without being absorbed. For that reason, it is best to chop the lettuce and other ingredients until they are finally small and easy to chew and swallow. Carrots and other vegetables can be grated. There are also kitchen gadgets that will chop, shred, etc., for you.

FAVORITE SOUPY SALAD

1 Romaine lettuce
5 tablespoons of olive oil
1 large or 2 small carrots grated
Juice of 1 large or 2 small, organic oranges, freshly
    squeezed
1/2 cup fresh carrot juice
1/2 cup cooked beets and beet juice
3 tablespoonfuls of Red Star Yeast mixed with
    herbal seasoning
Lemon juice or apple cider vinegar to taste

Chop the lettuce fine, then add all the other ingredients, and mix well.

If the salad is cold, warm slightly to room temperature. A large bowlful of this salad, with sliced, broiled potatoes, and half an avocado, makes a very delicious meal. Try it.

SALT SUBSTITUTES

There are many salt substitutes in the stores, but most of them contain some hidden salt, and should not be used. Instead, make your own seasoning, which is much better and less expensive.

BEVERAGES

Colas and the other soft drinks on the market are made with sugar, artificial coloring, artificial flavoring, and other chemicals that are harmful.

Alcoholic drinks are extremely bad in cases of arthritis. The slightest amount of alcohol will aggravate the pain of arthritis.

The best cool drinks are the *fresh* fruit and vegetable juices.

Coffee, sweetened with sugar, will keep arthritis going forever.

In another part of this book, you will find a number of pleasant-tasting coffee substitutes that are healthful. (They may not give the surge of energy that coffee does, but after you go on a natural diet, you will not require this unnatural stimulation, which is harmful. The caffeine in coffee is addictive.)

CONFECTIONS

Confections or sweets help to round out a balanced diet, but the ordinary cakes, candies, and other "junk" foods, made with sugar, cocoa, and chemicals, are not acceptable. Instead, you should use natural sweets, such as fresh fruits, dried fruits, and the cakes, cookies and other desserts given in this book.

Honey and dates are quite concentrated sweets and should be used sparingly. The fresh, sweet fruits are the best.

Often the fruits in the supermarkets are waxed and embalmed with biphenol and other chemicals. So try to get organic fruits, which have not been treated with chemicals.

SUGAR SUBSTITUTES

There are a number of these, but none are satisfactory. The only healthful items to use instead of refined sugar are honey, maple sugar, and unsulphured blackstrap molasses.

Some of the "maple sugar" syrups are mixed with sugar syrup. These should be avoided.

"Fructose" is very popular now. It is a white powder made from fruit, with all the nutrients removed. Although it comes from fruit, it is too highly concentrated, and an unnatural product. We do not recommend it.

LABELS

Again, we wish to stress the importance of reading the labels on your packaged foods. These are generally printed in very small letters, hard to read, so get a small pocket magnifying glass in the five and dime store, and use it. You will learn much and avoid trouble by reading the labels.

A WARNING ABOUT SOME SO-CALLED HEALTH FOODS

Such as tamari, miso, soy sauce, granola, yogurt, salt substitutes, sugar substitutes, and potato and corn chips:

All of the above products are quite popular with people who are trying to adhere to a healthful diet, but who do not realize that these items are really unhealthful. Let us see why.

Tamari, miso and soy sauce are loaded with salt, and are therefore very bad for arthritis, high blood pressure and other ailments. They should be strictly avoided.

CONCERNING POTATO CHIPS

Some of the health food stores carry potato chips that are made by frying in oil and grease which is used over and over. These *fried* chips are also seasoned with salt, and should not be used. A new corn chip is on the market which is *not fried*; instead, it is baked and salt-free. This product comes for the Garden of Eatin' company in Los Angeles. Look for it or ask for it at your local health food store.

CONCERNING GRANOLA

Granola is a sweet and tasty dry cereal food made with oats, honey, maple syrup, nuts, fruit and fruit juices. All are good ingredients, BUT the makers of this popular health food spoil it by ignorantly adding *salt*, which is not at all necessary.

CONCERNING BREWER'S YEAST

Beatrice Trum Hunter, one of today's foremost authorities on nutrition, disclosed this information: Some oil companies are promoting the sale of nutritional yeast which is made with petroleum products. These coal-tar products are cancer-forming and should be strictly avoided. So when buying Brewer's Yeast, make sure the brand you choose is *not* made from any petroleum products. We have found the Red Star brand satisfactory.

Brewer's Yeast is an important addition to the diet. It is a rich source of B vitamins, protein, and other essential nutrients.

CONCERNING NUTS AND SEEDS

The nuts* and seeds you use should be raw and unsalted. These foods are perishable and should be kept cool and in containers, especially during the warm, summer months. When you buy these perishable foods, carefully examine them to make sure they are not wormy. Also, taste them; they should taste good. If they don't, they are spoiled; take them back to the store and get a refund.

*Peanuts are legumes, not nuts, and so to lightly roast them is acceptable. Make sure they are not salted or roasted in oil.

WONDERFUL, HEALTHFUL GARLIC

The medical use of garlic goes back to ancient times. Modern man should use it more. The best way to use it is by pressing the cloves through a garlic press. Here are some of its benefits:

Garlic reduces serum cholesterol and triglyceride level (two blood fats that have been linked to an increased risk of heart attacks and atherosclerosis). There is clinical evidence to show that garlic dissolves globs of fat stuck in coronary arteries.

Garlic assists the body in dissolving existing clots and reducing the stickiness of the blood so more clots can't form.

Garlic reduces high blood pressure somewhat. It interferes with the transformation of normal cells into cancer cells.

Garlic protects cells against damage caused by oxidizing agents and heavy metal compounds that are common in modern industry.

Garlic boosts various immunological functions that can help the system fight cancer and Candida albicans, a yeast infection that afflicts millions of people.

SIX PAINLESS WAYS TO EAT LESS WITHOUT FEELING HUNGRY

1. Always eat breakfast. It gets your metabolism going at the beginning of the day.

2. Eat a mini-meal every three to fours throughout the day. You'll speed up your metabolism and stay full all the time.

3. Drink 12 cups of water every day; your stomach will stay fuller.

4. When you eat, choose more complex carbohydrates like pasta or vegetables. They make you feel fuller. Eat your salad first, then pasta and vegetables. Leave the fattening foods until last, when you are less hungry. High water content foods (such as juicy fruits, salads and vegetables) also make you feel fuller.

5. For times of the day when you're most likely to "blow it," plan activities that are not compatible with eating.

6. Before attending a party or other event when you are tempted to overeat, put on some tight clothes first.

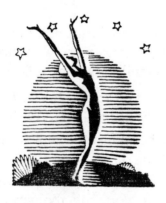

"Go forth under the open sky, and list
To Nature's teachings."

—William Cullen Bryant

CHAPTER XIX

RESULTS THAT COUNT

DR. STEPHEN GOITEIN
CHIROPRACTOR

(Specializing in Musculoskeletal Diseases)

Dear Doctors Welsh and Leonardo:

I have been recommending your book on arthritis to my patients who are suffering with this ailment. I am happy to report that <u>your plan really works</u>.

It is evident that you have uncovered the real cause of arthritis, and by removing this cause, you rid the patient of his or her ailment.

The price of your book is insignificant, compared with its value to anyone suffering with arthritis.

Sincerely,

Stephen Goitein, D. C.

Dr. Welsh!

Thanks to your plan to overcome arthritis, this old gal can now stoop without the thought, 'Maybe you won't get back up!' As my hips had it. And for me, that's something, as after 30 years of waitress and hostess work, these old legs have quite a few miles on them. YOUR PLAN IS GREAT!

Thankfully yours,

Helen Dunbar

A TRUE STORY OF PAIN AND SUFFERING, WITH A HAPPY ENDING!

Dear Doctors Welsh and Leonardo:

I am writing this letter because I feel it is the least I can do in the way of "thanks" for the improvement in my health, which started with the reading of your book, "FREEDOM FROM ARTHRITIS THROUGH NUTRITION."

I am 55 years old, and before reading your book I had suffered increasingly over a 15-year span. I made visits to a doctor specializing in arthritis from November, 1975, to November, 1977. He gave me a complete physical, x-rays included, and diagnosed my case as Psoriatic Arthritis. I took Indocin for quite some time, and also had two or three injections of Cortisone for the swelling in my fingers.

I did not get any noticeable good results. I stopped taking the Indocin on my own, because it didn't stop the pain, and it had bad aftereffects.

At the time, I did not know about your book, but I had read a few articles about faulty nutrition possibly causing some arthritic pain. But whenever I would try to discuss the subject with my doctor and showed him one of these articles, he just laughed about the whole subject.

Over a 15-year period, the pains crept up on me. The aches and pains were so bad that I couldn't wring the water from a washcloth. I couldn't hold a half-gallon of milk with one hand. I took a timer with me when I worked in the garden, because I would double up with pain if I worked longer than 20 minutes. I would fall into bed at night so full of aches and pains, and get up in the morning feeling the same way. The pains were over my whole body, from head to toe.

I purchased your book in September, 1979. By following your diet plan, I got FANTASTIC RESULTS! I began feeling better almost immediately, and have felt just great ever since. It is now June,

1980. I feel better than I have felt in many years, and can do more now than I could ten years ago!

All the above began with the reading of your book, and I am very grateful to you. What more can I say? You have my permission to use my information, if it can help someone else feel as good as I do.

Thanks again for your book, with your original Plan that Works! I don't know what I would have done without it.

Sincerely,
(Mrs.) June A. Hauser

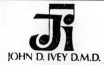

JOHN D. IVEY D.M.D.

I found your book easy to understand, informative, and very useful. It is a nutritional necessity in this age of over-processed food and unhealthy living. I will recommend it to my patients, whether they have arthritis or not, as nutrition affects our total body condition so strongly.

You have succeeded in providing a diet with recipes that will maintain a healthy body, and at the same time, be pleasant to the taste buds.

Thank you for your philosophy in making healthy living more enjoyable.

Dr. John D. Ivey, D.M.D.

Your book has been WORTH A MILLION DOLLARS TO ME! I can now walk much better. I work in my grocery store 40 hours a week. I thought I would be a cripple, but with your help, and God's, I can do almost anything now. May God bless you forevermore!

Edna V. Riley

After ordering your book, I put my 88-year-old mother on your program. In only TWO WEEKS, she reports that her very painful knee doesn't hurt anymore!

I am so glad that I sent for your book!

Myrtle Odin

A short time ago, I received your revolutionary book on arthritis. My 26-year-old daughter has had rheumatoid arthritis for five years. After following the instructions in your book, she is now feeling much better. She is able to go shopping again, as her ankle swelling is gone. The swelling in her wrists and fingers is also greatly relieved. Many thanks to both you authors.

Your book, which is really a comprehensive health manual, includes a plan which means wonderful relief for arthritis sufferers.

Sincerely and gratefully yours,
Adrian Middelkoop

Dear Friends:
I cannot thank you enough for your book on arthritis. I have followed your plan, and am very happy with the results. Since following your plan, I have lost 30 pounds. I haven't been to a doctor for two years, and I feel great!

When I think of the pain I went through! Your book is truly a great blessing. I would be happy to recommend it to anyone.

Thanking you again, and God Bless You!

Dominick Ali

Recently, while visiting my mother, I noticed the remarkable improvement she has shown since adopting your program. So, since I was troubled with arthritis, I decided to adopt your plan also.

In a short time, I experienced increased energy and vitality, a clearer and smoother skin and a tremendous sense of health and well being. In addition, I lost some of my excess weight, even though I ate plenty of food.

So, you can see that I am an enthusiastic convert and most eager to commend you both for presenting such a basic and comprehensive plan, in your book on arthritis and health in general.

I no longer have any arthritis pain! I do not hesitate to recommend your book to anyone and everyone.

Gratefully yours,
Riki Wells

———————

Your book on arthritis means more to me than words can say. The recipes in the book are priceless. To my knowledge, they are unavailable from any other source.

I am so happy that you wrote the book that I want to thank you for sharing with me, and all who read the book, your profound knowledge on the subject of health.

Sincerely,
Helen R. Smith

———————

I enjoyed reading your book on arthritis, because I learned a lot I didn't know. I am following your plan, and I am feeling much better now. I had arthritis in my hands, arms, shoulders, hips, legs and feet. I could not walk without a limp, but now I am walking much better, and I can use my hands and arms much better.

I am going to keep following your plan, so I can feel good the rest of my life. Thanks so very much for your help. I wish you the best of everything. May God Bless you for helping humanity!

Gratefully,

Margaret Boggs

(Note: Mrs. Boggs wrote this letter ONLY 18 DAYS AFTER RECEIVING THE BOOK!)

After only one month of following your prescribed diet, I feel so wonderful I can't resist writing a note of thanks.

For years I had arthritis in my right shoulder, elbow, wrist, and in both hands. But NO MORE! The stiffness and pain are gone. I am able to knit, crochet, and practice on my piano. These are activities I thought I would never again enjoy. My complexion is clear. I have shed ten unwanted pounds, and am enjoying the most delightful meals I have ever eaten.

My family joins me in thanking you for starting my on this healthful program, for they, too, have benefited from your book.

I will be 56 years old on June 2nd, but I feel younger and healthier every day!

Sincerely,
Margaret Otterson

Dear Doctors/Authors:

If any of the following can help the readers of your book, feel free to use it.

I had bursitis of my left shoulder. The medical doctor offered no suggestions, except to take pills. I play classical guitar, and it was getting to a point where I couldn't hold my left arm up for more than a few minutes at a time, and I was seriously considering giving up the guitar.

Then I started having pain in my right shoulder. That's when I got panicky, and wrote you for help. I read your book and immediately started on your diet.

In about three weeks, I noticed a remarkable improvement. My arms and shoulder no longer ached like a toothache. I was able to continue playing the guitar.

Thank you so much for your book, and I hope that others who have this problem or a similar one, will try your plan for a few weeks. IT REALLY DOES WORK!

Sincerely,
Avis Barnes

For five years, I was having pain in my back, elbows, arms, and fingers. The pain got so bad these last two years that I couldn't walk, sit or stand. I would fall if I did not hold on to a chair or wall. I sent for your book and thought I would give it a try.

In two months, I was much better. NOW, I HAVE NO PAIN!

It's wonderful to be free from pain and walk without having to hold on to chairs and walls. My husband can sleep at night without hearing me cry for help. I do all my housework without pain. I feel younger and healthier.

Thank you, both, for your book and method that has given me blessed relief, after five years of suffering!

I am one who knew pain, but who is now free from pain.

Gratefully,
Lynn Livingston

The world-famous author, WILL DURANT, who wrote the book *The Story of Philosophy* and the 11-volume work (with his wife Ariel), *The Story of Civilization*, wrote to the authors of the book on arthritis, as follows:

I have just finished reading your splendid book. I am enclosing my check for the very reasonable charge for the work that went into the publishing the book in its convenient format.

I shall try to follow faithfully all your patient counsel.

I applaud your work, and you may, if you wish, quote me. Bless you and your aides. I hope a hundred million people will read your book and obey it.

Yours gratefully,

Will Durant

Dear Doctors Welsh and Leonardo:

I am ordering three copies of your new edition of FREEDOM FROM ARTHRITIS THROUGH NUTRITION. I have an older edition of the book, which I have used for years. I feel it has helped me so much that I wanted to get the updated edition for myself, and give one copy to a friend with Berger's Disease.

I feel that this book should be read by the younger people, before they get some of these illnesses. Thank you for writing the book. It is nice to know there are people who really care.

Best regards,

Steve Stephenson

I want to thank you from the bottom of my heart for your program that seemingly, by some magical power, causes one's pain and complications to disappear. Please accept my sincere appreciation for your help.

O. Nygren

I am dropping you this note to let you know that I feel much better, and have no more pains in my hands, legs, and shoulder. I also have lost a little weight. I do thank you very much for your wonderful book on arthritis. God bless you.

(Mrs.) Victoria Forsythe

I do not have arthritis, but ordered your book to help friends who have it. When I read your book, I realized that this is the most sensible book on arthritis that I have ever read — and I have read plenty of them.

One of my friends is following the plan, and the pain in her knee has left her.

May God bless you in what you are doing for others.

Sincerely,

Lorna M. Benton

Your book has been worth a million dollars to me! I thought I would be a cripple, but with your plan, I can do almost everything now. God bless you both for writing this wonderful book.

(Mrs.) Roberta Edwards

What a pleasure it was to receive your splendid book on arthritis! I am proving the thoroughness and accuracy of your advice. I like it. I know IT WORKS!

Sincerely,
Mildred D. Emrick

I have not had any attacks of arthritis since I received your book. I followed your plan, and know that my changed diet is the reason for my good health lately. I am 77 years old, and do quite a bit of hard work. I am a farmer. Thank you so much for sharing your valuable health knowledge with the public.

Albert Hieb

Thank you for the fantastic book you have sent me. I will share it and tell others about it.
We are following your plan, and it is helping us very much.
May God bless you many times over.

Sincerely yours,
Charles Meyer

I am so happy to have found your book. Now I AM FREE FROM PAIN, and am enjoying life with my family and friends. I hope that my letter can help many people who have given up hope. There is always hope, and prayers are answered. Now I am free, and a very happy person.

Linda Laymon

Here is an order for another copy of your wonderful book on arthritis. Since last month, when I bought my first copy, I have been so sold on it, that I have been telling all my friends about it. I am really sold on your plan.

P.S. I made the honey-carrot cake according to your recipe. It was delicious!

(Mrs.) Donna Andrews

At the time I sent for your book, my hands were terribly sore. I take care of the bookkeeping for my husband's business, and writing was very painful.

Now I am just fine, even though I have not followed the plan 100%.

My husband went on the diet with me. We have both lost ten or more pounds, and my husband feels better than he has in many years.

Your diet plan is fabulous! Thanks!

Bertha Doolittle

I received your book just about three weeks ago, and am finding it very helpful. Your original recipes are great!

I lent your book to a friend who is troubled with shoulder pains. I am trying to faithfully go by your book. I think it is wonderful, and I want to thank you for writing it.

Sincerely,
(Mrs.) Michelle Erwin

I am following your plan, and am delighted. Before I got your book, I used drugs for years to alleviate the pain. I also spent much money on acupuncture, with no help. So you can understand why I feel so happy with your plan, which is really getting results.

Sincerely yours,
Frances Roberts

JESSE MERCER GEHMAN, N.D., D.C., M.N.
Consulting Health Specialist

Dear Doctors Welsh and Leonardo:

You did a superlative piece of writing in producing your book on arthritis. The book teems with essentials which are so clearly and forthrightly presented that none can misinterpret them.

The beauty of your book is that it serves the dual purpose of being a specific treatment for arthritis and at the same time is a comprehensive nutritional guidebook. It deserves the attention of any person seriously interested in achieving health and well being. All in all, you have produced an unparalleled health book.

It is not only for the usual health seeker, but should be a MUST for physicians, nutritionists, nurses and public educators.

Very sincerely,

Jesse Mercer Gehman

I have read and re-read your very well-written book on arthritis. You have presented your plan in a manner that everyone can understand and follow.

You are doing a great service for humanity by producing this marvelous manual. Keep up the good work.

Sincerely yours,

Nathan A. Styrt, D.D.S., F.A.G.D.

Dear Doctors Welsh and Leonardo:

About a month ago, Mrs. Foster, an elderly, ailing lady, asked me to take a position in her home to prepare healthful meals for her, and also help her cope with her crippling arthritis.

I heard about your book, sent for it, and immediately began to apply the simple instructions in the book, in order to help Mrs. Foster with her terrible pain.

Well, I can't begin to tell you the change that came over this woman within a period of TWO WEEKS! Her closed fingers opened, and her constant pain subsided seemingly miraculously. She was a changed woman. We were both thrilled with the results. She had gotten relief from pain in her body for the first time in years, all because of the wonderful health plan in your book. She calls your truly amazing book her "bible." I am writing this letter to express our sincere gratitude.

Healthfully yours,

Mary Gae

I had Rheumatoid Arthritis for 19 years; I was under the care of a rheumatologist all this time. I took every drug from Prednisone to Indocin.

I was looking for a nutritionist with your knowledge, for a long time.

Your book arrived on May 1. I felt improvement after two weeks on your plan. Now it's been almost nine weeks, and I am feeling much better. I expect to continue on your plan as long as I live.

Sincerely,

Edythe Axelrod

Dear Sirs:

Recently I purchased your book on arthritis. My need was great, as I have been a victim of anemia, arthritis and rheumatism for years. But now I am well on the road to recovery by doing as you suggest in your book.

I am planning to write an article for my local paper, "How I Have Been Helped with my Arthritis". I would like to share this important knowledge with others.

Sincerely yours,

Theresa Thornton

Last week I received your book on arthritis, and started on your proper eating plan, I have already noticed a difference in the arthritis in my knees. The pain is subsiding, and I am very happy, thanks to your book.

You may use my letter as a testimonial. I am pleased and honored to have you include me with the rest of the happy people who have been helped by your book.

Sincerely yours,

(Mrs.) Rose Gallagher

Dear Dr. Welsh

I Am 13 years old And I had Rheumatiod Arthritis. I read your book Freedom from Arthritis Through Nutrition. I followed the diet And I was freed from my Arthritis.

I had Arthritis since January 21, 1980. I read your book in May 1980 And by the end of May I was free from Arthritis.

Thank You

Your friend
Mia Kirk ♥

CHAPTER XX

THE ASCENDING STEPS IN A PURIFIED DIET .
LONGEVITY WITHOUT SENILITY.
THE "GREAT SECRET."

by Dr. Bianca Leonardo

Dear Reader:

If you want to look youthful, although on in years, if you want to be slender, and have good teeth into an advanced age — if you want *longevity with super health and great energy* instead of aches, pains, disease, and resort to drugs and surgery — in other words, if you desire the true "fountain of youth," read on.

The cure for most physical problems is not in the doctor's office, the hospital, or the pharmacy; it is in *your kitchen*. Yes, you are what you eat.

We have given you many delicious vegetarian recipes in this book. For a person who is on a typical meat diet, with all its fat, cholesterol, and polluting qualities, it may be a giant step to "go vegetarian." But, truly, that is the first step.

There are further steps, or stages of advancement, I want to tell you about, for your consideration. Many years of study and experience have gone into this chapter.

Let us take an average American, whom we will call "Mr./Ms. A. A." Men and women are, of course, in the same situation when it comes to diet. For smooth writing, I will use the pronouns "he and his" rather than the cumbersome form "he/she", "his/hers." Ladies, please excuse, and include yourselves.

He eats many of his meals at MacDonald's, or another fast food eatery; hamburgers are his daily fare. He also takes alcohol in one or more of its various forms. (He may also take tobacco smoke into his lungs, but we will write only about food and drink here.)

Mr. A. A. gives little thought to the quality of the foods that he takes into his belly, whether they are good for him or not. Aren't they advertised everywhere — on television, on billboards, in newspapers and magazines? Don't celebrities (the American gods and goddesses whom the public worships) endorse them?

But, one day, our average American reads something — like this book, or another health book, or perhaps an article in a magazine. (The information is everywhere today; national health organizations, doctors, and nutritionists are sending it out constantly.)

THIS STARTS MR. A. A. THINKING! He gets the bright and right idea that perhaps the scientists are RIGHT, and that the hamburger companies, the dairy companies, etc., are WRONG — that *they have a vested interest in selling him their products for profit* — *they care not for his health!* His eyes, tightly closed up to now, begin to open. His brain cells begin to work. A desire stirs in him to learn more. Perhaps it is time to stop being a "couch potato." Television is his only form of recreation, unless it is stopping at a bar for a drink, on the way home from work.

Perhaps he is grossly overweight. He cannot help but notice the stares of others when he passes. It is embarrassing when he cannot fit into a single seat on a plane or bus or in a movie theatre. He has heard that such overweight is hard on his heart, and that he will have a short life.

A desire to lose his excess weight increases. He thinks: "How I would love to ride a bicycle again, or a horse, or go ballroom dancing, or square dancing."

Finally willing to face up to the facts, he determines to do something about the gnawing realization that he must pursue another track. He has only to overcome the force of habit, overcome his addictive food style, and embark on a course of health. Sufficient desire will do it. There is an abundance of information available everywhere — in government reports, on public service videos, in magazines on the newsrack at the supermarket, and in books, like this one.

Here are the five steps one can take — from the bottom rung of the ladder of ill health and overweight — to the top, of the ideal we described in our first paragraph — super health and energy. All those in the natural health movement have gone this route. Sometimes it takes years to take all five steps, but the important thing is to *start*. You may stop on any rung of this ladder of health, where you feel comfortable.

STEP ONE

Discontinue the consumption of all red meat. That means, if you still frequent one of the fast food eateries, you will eat from the salad bar, or find a non-red-meat entree. It is far better to eat at home. Take as many meals at home as possible. There you have total control over what goes into your body.

STEP TWO

Mr. A. A. is now reading about health, and learning about foods that are harmful to his health. During Step Two, he learns that chickens are very diseased and full of harmful drugs, as are the red meat animals. He deletes chicken from his diet.

STEP THREE

Mr. A. A. learns more, and his desire increases to purify his diet. He researches the subject of fish. Once fish was the best of flesh foods, but not it is not so. The waters wherein they live are polluted with mercury, waste from factories, etc., and the fish are diseased. Also, fish is the most perishable of flesh foods, and it is impossible to get them fresh enough. One would have to fish for them himself, in the wilderness where the waters are relatively unpolluted, to get fresh fish.

Mr. A. A. deletes fish and seafood from his diet. He is now a vegetarian. He may stay on this step of the ladder for a long time, or, if he learns more and wants to go further, he may advance to Step 4.

STEP FOUR

Mr. A. A. hears about the "vegan" movement. Vegans are people who do not use animal by-products, namely, milk, cheese, and eggs. He is really thinking now. If the animals are diseased and full of harmful drugs, then their products, namely, milk from the cow and eggs from the chicken, would be likewise, would they not? He is striving to learn the true facts about health, and has the discipline to lead him to the ideal diet. He now reads vegetarian and vegan literature, joins an organization, and attends conventions to learn more.

One of the books Mr. A. A. has read is *Diet for a New America*, by John Robbins, a 1987 Pulitzer Prize nominee. (Actually, a better title would be *Diet for a New World*, for the entire Western world has the same diet patterns and same health problems that America has. Food is a world problem, as all nations are now inter-related.)

In this book, the entire meat question is thoroughly explored. Mr. A. A. learns that animal flesh and animal by-products are not only harmful to his health, but also injurious to our fragile and over-burdened planet. In fact, animal breeding and consumption is already becoming the main cause of a totally unlivable planet, as well as famine and starvation for people of Third World countries. There is, in addition, the problem of the billions of dollars the U. S. is spending on "disease care" annually. (*It is not health care*, which would be teaching the prevention of disease, and nutrition.) Together with other national waste, these billions can bankrupt our nation.

It is widely believed that infirmity and degenerative diseases are natural accompaniments of advanced years. THIS IS NOT SO. People of all ages can be in good health until it is time to "make the transition." This writer knows a number of such persons; what one can do, all can do, if there is sufficient knowledge and motivation.

STEP FIVE

THE GREAT SECRET

Mr. A. A. is now a vegan, and on the plus side of the problem. He has lost weight, and has youthful vigor. He notices, that after dining, if he should happen to eat only living foods (sometimes called raw foods) — fresh fruits, fresh vegetables, seeds, nuts, and sprouted grains, he feels so much better!

So, gradually, he begins to delete some of the cooked foods he has been eating, replacing them with *living* foods. He eats mostly at home, but if he does dine out, he is careful about the restaurant and the meal he selects.

The greater percentage of living foods (especially organic), the more healthful the diet. There are so many advantages, namely:

(a) Better health and more energy;

(b) Lower food bills, as well as gas/electric bills (that portion used for cooking);

(c) Much time saved. Fewer dishes to wash and less time to prepare meals.

(d) It is easy to overeat with cooked foods. With living foods, that must be chewed, it is natural and easy to eat just the right amount.

FOUR GREAT ONES ON LIVING FOODS

(I, Dr. Leonardo, knew or know three of these persons.

Dr. Wigmore and Mrs. Hazel S. Richards are still alive.)

To encourage you to go this far (Step 5 on the ladder of Super Health), I will acquaint you with four wise ones, who were or are Living Food devotees. There are many others in the Living Food movement.

I. Dr. Norman Walker

Dr. Norman W. Walker (who had earned six college degrees: M.D., D.O., D.C., N.D., D.Sc., and Ph.D.) was not only a brilliant man, but a humanitarian. He had more than knowledge — he had wisdom, and knew how to live. He proved that by living to the age of 109 years, working to the end. He left this plane on June 6, 1985, as the result of an accident. Good, kind, humane, selfless, wise, he was one of a kind. (A letter from him to me, follows this chapter.)

II. Dr. Ann Wigmore

I call her "sproutarian, humanitarian." Whenever you see sprouts in a supermarket, salad bar or elsewhere, you can thank her. She made sprouting popular. "Ann Wigmore is to sprouts what George Washington Carver was to peanuts." (Vegetarian Times.)

Dr. Wigmore spent much time in India, selflessly helping and teaching these people, showing them they can have a nourishing diet for pennies, instead of lacking food. This poor nation cannot support traditional foods like meat, for its teeming multi-millions of population. The people can produce some of their own foods, and without land, by sprouting at home.

She now has two institutes where Westerners go to learn more — one in Boston, and one in Puerto Rico. She is a dear friend, whom I often had as a speaker when I was Founder/ President of Vegetarian Society, Inc., in the Los Angeles area, for 15 years. She is now 83, vigorous, slender, still working and teaching others. (See Chapter V.)

III. Mrs. Vera Richter

She was a present-day living example of the value of a living food diet. At the age of 79, she ran a one-half acre farm in the city of Los Angeles. She had a youthful appearance, worked barefooted in her garden, slept outdoors, and enjoyed the products of the soil which her labors had enriched. (The most nourishment comes from organic fruits and vegetables, freshly picked.) She wrote a "Cook-less Book," with recipes using living foods.

I am using the term "living foods" instead of "raw foods." Not only is it a more appealing term, it is *true* term. Meat can be called "raw," but cannot be called "living." In fact, it is as dead as a corpse, and is exactly that — part of the corpse of a dead animal. Plant foods were designed by God, through Mother Nature, God's expression for mankind's sustenance.

Those people who can grow their own fruits and vegetables, eating them immediately after removing them from their mother plant, are indeed fortunate.

One lady who grows her own told me that her health has improved tremendously since she started growing her food. With her, the time is short between the fruit or vegetables leaving their life force connection, and her eating it.

Mankind's original, true, natural, and wholesome diet is outlined in the first chapter of Genesis (1:29):

"And God said, Behold, I have given you every herb bearing seed, which is upon the face of all the earth, and every tree, in which is the fruit of a tree yielding seed; to you it shall be for meat (food.)"

IV. MRS. HAZEL S. RICHARDS

Recently I met this wonderful and inspiring lady, who was born June 11, 1902. (90 in 1992.) She was a pupil of Dr. Ann Wigmore, and worked at her institute in Boston years ago. Now, Mrs. Richard's diet is about 85% "living food." She lives in her own home in a senior community in Southern California, and drives some of the other senior citizens to their doctor appointments, but has no need for any such visits herself!

Her teaching is in a book entitled *Learn the True Science of Perfect Health, with Recipes that Work*. She states: "Remember: You can only build perfect health in an unpolluted body."

* * * * *

My thanks, appreciation and honors to these four great ones,* who have lived/are living what they know to be the truth — that "living foods" are the best for health. This diet is the diet of the "Garden of Eden," a blissful time when there was no killing, but mankind sustained itself on the fruits and other plants provided by Mother Nature. Even though many of us now live in cities, we can still feed ourselves this way. Living Foods are a humane diet, too. There is no killing for our food. It is not necessary.

*There are many other persons, past and present, we know, whom we could honor.

Dear Reader, I urge you to follow the Wisdom of these Pioneers who are showing us the best way to live.

However, that is not all there is to say on this subject. One must not indulge in any of the "baddies" — caffeine drinks, alcohol, or tobacco. One must ESCHEW ALL DRUGS. Legal or illegal, the body does not know the difference. Finally, diet — even of all natural foods — is not all there is to health. THERE ARE SEVEN LAWS IN HEALTH EACH OF WHICH MUST BE OBEYED. They are: Fresh Air; Natural Food; Exercise; Water (Internal and External Uses); Sunshine; Sleep and Rest; The Mental/Spiritual: prayer, meditation, cheerfulness, doing good deeds, (giving of yourself, selflessness), positive thinking, etc.

Those practicing these natural health laws find their need for doctors disappearing. Prevention is much of the answer. If a problem does occur, they either fast and let the body heal itself (as animals do), or get help from a holistic (drugless) doctor.

This is the complete package — Nature's Laws, of which mankind is so largely ignorant. Obey them, and you can look forward to longevity without senility — a long life of usefulness and happiness. God Bless You and Keep you in Health! But you must do your part.

All four wise ones have written books on this "Living Food Lifestyle," and these books are available through this publisher.* Or ask your health food store.

* Tree of Life Publications,   P.O. Box 126,   Joshua Tree, CA 92252
    (A book catalog is $1.00.)

A LETTER FROM DR. NORMAN W. WALKER
to Bianca Leonardo

Dear Dr. Leonardo:

Thank you for the copy of your book, *Cancer and Other Diseases Caused by Meat Consumption* — *Here's the Evidence.* I hope you will sell a million of these.

As you no doubt know, I am not in favor of meat, even at its best, as a source of protein. In addition, there is the esthetic angle, or rather, the lack thereof.

People fail to realize that the body needs only an average of three of four ounces of protein replenishment a day. Nitrogen is its important ingredient. Where do we get it?

Almighty God KNEW how much we need and its best regular source, namely, the AIR WE BREATHE! It contains 75% nitrogen and we get a mouthful, or nose-full, with every breath! Raw vegetables, fruits and sprouted seeds supply the balance.

I again thank you for your book and for the message you expound.

With my kindest regards and best wishes,

Sincerely yours,

N.W. Walker, M.D., D.O., D.C., N.D., D.Sc., Ph.D.

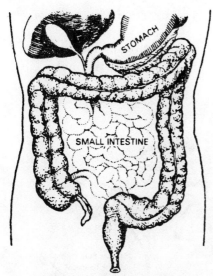

ABOVE: What a person's Colon should be.

BADLY DISTORTED COLON:

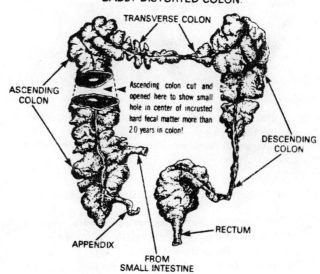

TRANSVERSE COLON

ASCENDING COLON

Ascending colon cut and opened here to show small hole in center of incrusted hard fecal matter more than 20 years in colon!

DESCENDING COLON

RECTUM

APPENDIX

FROM SMALL INTESTINE

Credit: *The Natural Way to Vibrant Health,* by
Dr. Norman W. Walker

This is the ascending colon, with solid impaction of fecal matter. There is only a tiny hole clear, in the center.

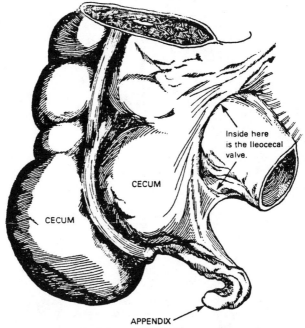

This illustrates the lower part of the ascending colon, showing the appendix and the ileocaecal valve within the junction of the small intestine with the ascending colon.

The ileocaecal valve is equipped with a safety mechanism which opens automatically to let matter pass through from the small intestine into the colon, but closes automatically to prevent any substance, liquid or solid, from returning into or entering into the small intestine from the colon. But if this does happen, you are in trouble.

HEALTH REPORTS/LITERATURE

1. Correct Food Combining
2. Spiritual Healing
3. Vaccinations Do Not Protect
4. Recommended Reading (Health Book List)
5. Health Spas (List)
6. Colonic Therapists (List); A source for the colemic board.
7. Fasting Institutions;
   Natural Health Organizations (Lists)
8. Source of Organic Foods (List)
9. Candida (Yeast Overgrowth —
   80 million Americans suffer from it.)
10. Book Catalog from Tree of Life Publications
11. Highlights of best seller *Diet for a New America*

Women's Topics

12. "The Pill"
13. Why Nurse Your Baby?
14. The Hidden Horrors of Hysterectomy

15. HEALTH VIDEOS: (see next page)

Highlights of 10 recommended Health Videos, and
How to Order Them

TITLES:

(1) Eat Smart
(2) Lower Your Cholesterol Now
(3) Fit or Fat for the '90's
(4) Fit for Life
(5) Fit for Life Delicious Vegetable Entrees
(6) Friendly Foods — Gourmet Vegetarian
   (Bro. Ron Picarski, chef.)
(7) Mouthwatering Meatless Meals
(8) Healthy, Wealthy, and Wise — Vegetarian Lifestyle
(9) Health Through Living Foods (Dr. Ann Wigmore)
(10) Diet for a New America (John Robbins)

— —

Order from:

TREE OF LIFE PUBLICATIONS
P. O. Box 126
Joshua Tree, CA, 92252

$11.00 for all 15 Items — or select 6 for $6.00
(postage, any tax included)

CHAPTER XXII

Other Titles Published by Tree of Life Publications

P. O. Box 126, Joshua Tree, CA 92252

Also, charge or mail orders from BookMasters, 800-247-6553

1. *They Conquered AIDS! True Life Adventures,*
   by Scott J. Gregory, O.M.D. and Bianca Leonardo, N.D.
   Hard cover, 360 pages, $19.95 (Reduced price.)
   Called "the most inspiring book of our generation."

2. *Conquering AIDS Now with Natural Therapies,*
   by Gregory and Leonardo, $12.95. (Now a Warner book)

3. *How to Conquer Cancer Naturally,*
   by Johanna Brandt, N.D. $9.95
   Dr. Brandt had phenomenal success with cancer patients,
   using her natural diet plan, in the U. S. and in her native
   South Africa.

4. *Adventures in Kinship with All Life,*
   by J. Allen Boone, $9.95. (The sequel to the best-selling
   Kinship With All Life.) Inspirational.

5. *The Unknown Life of Jesus Christ,*
   by N. Notovich. Based on a document in a Tibetan
   lamasery, explaining the 18 "lost years" of Jesus between
   the ages of 12 and 30. Price, $10.00.

Add shipping:
   $2.00, one book; $2.50, two books;
   $3.00 for 3 to 5 books.
   Californians, please add appropriate sales tax.

PART II
RECIPES

Zelda
Son Nov 7 TNT